Clinics in

Obstetrics and Gynaecology

QUESTIONS and ANSWERS

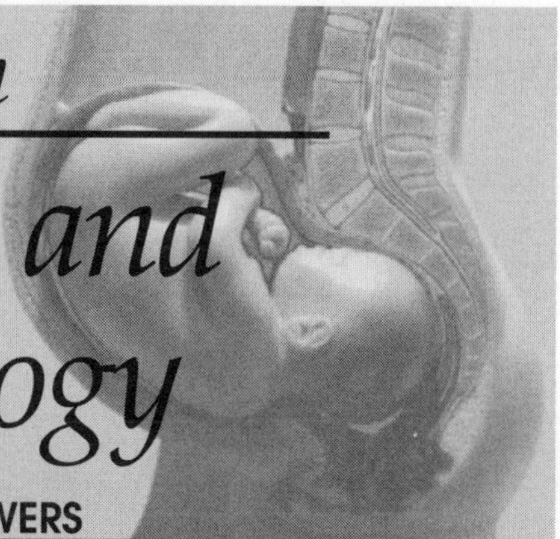

CBS Clinics in ... Series

Series Editor

SABYASACHI SIRCAR MD MAMS
Professor of Physiology
University College of Medical Sciences, Delhi

Clinics in

Obstetrics and Gynaecology

QUESTIONS and ANSWERS

AMITA SUNEJA
MD FICMCH FICOG MNAMS
Professor, Department of Obstetrics and Gynaecology
University College of Medical Sciences and
Guru Teg Bahadur Hospital
Delhi

RASHMI MALIK
MBBS MD
Junior Specialist
Department of Obstetrics and Gynaecology
Guru Teg Bahadur Hospital
Delhi

CBS

CBS Publishers & Distributors Pvt Ltd

New Delhi • Bengaluru • Pune • Kochi • Chennai

Clinics in
Obstetrics and Gynaecology
Questions and Answers

ISBN: 978-81-239-1984-3

First Edition: 2011

Published by Satish Kumar Jain and produced by Vinod K. Jain for
CBS Publishers & Distributors Pvt Ltd
4819/XI Prahlad Street, 24 Ansari Road, Daryaganj,
New Delhi 110 002, India.
Ph: 23289259, 23266861, 23266867
Fax: 011-23243014
Website: www.cbspd.com
e-mail: delhi@cbspd.com
cbspubs@vsnl.com
cbspubs@airtelmail.in.

Branches

- Bengaluru: Seema House 2975, 17th Cross, K.R. Road, Banasankari 2nd Stage, Bengaluru 560 070, Karnataka
  Ph: +91-80-26771678/79 Fax: +91-80-26771680 e-mail: bangalore@cbspd.com
- Pune: Bhuruk Prestige, Sr. No. 52/12/2+1+3/2 Narhe, Haveli (Near Katraj-Dehu Road Bypass), Pune 411 051, Maharashtra
  Ph: 020-64704058, 64704059, 32342277 Fax: +91-020-24300160 e-mail: pune@cbspd.com
- Kochi: 36/14 Kalluvilakam, Lissie Hospital Road, Kochi 682 018, Kerala
  Ph: +91-484-4059061-65 Fax: +91-484-4059065 e-mail: cochin@cbspd.com
- Chennai: 20, West Park Road, Shenoy Nagar, Chennai 600 030, Tamil Nadu
  Ph: +91-44-26260666, 26208620 Fax: +91-44-45530020 email: chennai@cbspd.com

Printed at Manipal Press Limited, Manipal, Karnataka

Foreword

It gives me immense pleasure to welcome this wonderful book authored by my colleagues who are dedicated and inspirational teachers. This book is one of its own kinds consisting of clinical case discussions along with questions and answers. This will stimulate the students to tailor the textbook knowledge to the clinical situations. The book offers interesting and thought-provoking material to tingle the young minds. The information is clinically relevant and simple, therefore when learnt in this manner is likely to stick for long.

The best part of this book is that it is written by only two authors so that you will find consistency of ideas throughout the book. The book should be of great interest to both the undergraduate and postgraduate students. Even resident doctors and general practitioners will benefit from it. My compliments to the authors and the editor who have done a great service by rekindling the enjoyment during learning of the subject.

Neelam B Vaid MBBS MD FICOG
Director-Professor and Head
Department of Obstetrics and Gynaecology
University College of Medical Sciences and GTB Hospital
Delhi

Preface

It was in the summer of 2007 that I requested Amita to write a book on Obstetrics and Gynaecology. Both of us had graduated from Maulana Azad Medical College, New Delhi, and Amita was a year senior to me. She was the topper of her batch while I always found the going tough, especially with the practical examinations in clinical subjects. Years later, with several years of teaching experience behind me, I knew why I found the practical examinations difficult despite being thorough in theory. I realized that to make sense of the clinics, undergraduates require a very different book. In medical subjects, the syllabus is defined rather fuzzily and by far, the most clearly-defined syllabus springs from the constellation of patients that throng a busy hospital. By the same token, the most appropriate book for undergraduate medical students has to be the transcript of the clinical routine and its raison d'être.

Why could not there be a book that focused only on what is taught in the clinics? Why can not the book contain the answers to all the queries of the student? It was precisely with these two questions that I approached Amita three years ago. "Please write a book", I requested her, "On what you mostly do in the clinics and why you do so". Writing the book on *'what to do–and why'* turned out to be a task more formidable than we presumed initially and after several months, Amita invited Rashmi to help her out. I contributed to the book a barrage of questions–very basic questions that only the naïve mind could ask. I also made numerous suggestions on rephrasing the answers to make them crisp, easily comprehensible, and relevant to the questions posed, while the authors, in fitness of things, had the final say.

Although this is a question-answer book that should prove useful to the undergraduate students in the clinics as well as in examinations, it is fundamentally different from the other books in the market with similar titles that list the *viva voce* questions that are commonly asked by the examiners and the answers expected of the students. On the contrary, this book lists the questions that are likely to be asked by an inquisitive student and the answers that a consultant would provide. Unlike the other books, the number and type of questions in this book will never be limited by the examiners' repertoire but shall continue to draw sustenance from the endless stream of naïve queries of the students. I would therefore request the readers to mail their questions to *qlinics@gmail.com* and thereby contribute to making this book better with every edition.

Sabyasachi Sircar MD MAMS
Professor of Physiology
University College of Medical Sciences, Delhi

Preface

Contents

GYNAECOLOGY

Abbreviations

A/B	Antibiotics
AC	Abdominal circumference
ACA	Anticardiolipin antibodies
ACE	Angiotensin-converting enzyme
AFB	Acid fast bacilli
AFI	Amniotic fluid index
AFV	Amniotic fluid volume
AIS	Androgen insensitivity syndrome
ANC	Antenatal care
APH	Antepartum hemorrhage
APS	Antiphospholipid antibody syndrome
ARM	Artificial rupture of membranes
ART	Assisted reproductive technology
ASA	Acetyl salicylic acid
ASCUS	Atypical squamous cells of unknown significance
AUB	Abnormal uterine bleeding
AV	Anteverted
AZT	Azidothymidine
BG	Blood group
BMI	Body mass index
BOH	Bad obstetric history
BOM	Bag of membranes
BP	Blood pressure
BPD	Biparietal diameter
BPP	Biophysical profile
BPS	Biophysical profile scoring
BPT	Biparietal diameter
BSO	Bilateral salpingo-oophorectomy
BT, CT	Bleeding time, clotting time
c/s	Culture and sensitivity
CA-125	Cancer antigen-125
CBC	Complete blood count
CI	Clinical Impression
COC	Combined oral contractive
CPD	Cephalopelvic disproportion
CRL	Crown-rump length
CRT	Clot retraction time
CST	Continue same therapy
Cx	Cervix
D & C	Dilatation and curettage
DFMR	Daily fetal movement rate
DHT	Dihydrotestosterone
DIC	Disseminated intravascular coagulation
DNS	Dextrose normal saline
DO	Detrusor overactivity
DOTS	Directly observed treatment shortcourse
DTA	Deep transverse arrest
DUB	Dysfunctional uterine bleeding
DVT	Deep vein thrombosis
EB	Endometrial biopsy
EDD	Expected date of delivery
EFW	Estimated fetal weight
ERT	Estrogen replacement therapy
ET	Endometrial thickness
FA	Folic acid
FGR	Fetal growth restriction
FHS	Fetal heart sound
FL	Femur length
FPP	Fetal parts palpable
FS	Fersolate
FSH	Follicle stimulating hormone
FTNVD	Full term normal vaginal delivery
FTVD	Full term vaginal delivery
Fx	Fornix
GA	General anesthesia
GC	General condition
GCT	Glucose challenge test
GDM	Gestational diabetes mellitus
GSI	Genuine stress incontinence
GTN	Gestational trophoblastic neoplasia
H/o, h/o	history of
HAART	Highly active antiretroviral therapy
HSA	Husband's semen analysis
Hb	Hemoglobin

HBsAg Hepatitis B surface antigen
HC Head circumference
HELLP Hemolysis, elevated liver enzymes, low platelet count
HOPI History of present illness
HOPP History of present pregnancy
HPE Histopathological examination
HRT Hormone replacement therapy
HSG Hysterosalpingography
HVS High vaginal swab
HWY Hundred women years
ICS International continence society
ICSI Intracytoplasmic sperm injection
ICU Intensive care unit
IR Insulin resistance
IUCD Intrauterine contraceptive device
IUD Intrauterine death
IUD Intrautrine device
IUGR Intrauterine growth restriction
IUI Intrauterine insemination
IVF *In vitro* fertilization
IVF-ET *In vivo* fertilization and embryo transfer
IVP Intravenous pyelography
KFT Kidney function test
KUB Kidney, ureter, bladder
L/E Local examination
LA Lupus anticoagulant
LEEP Loop electrosurgical excision procedure
LFT Liver function test
LH Luteinizing hormone
LMP Last menstrual period
LNG-IUS Nevonorgestrel intrauterine system
LOA Left occiput anterior
LPD Luteal phase defects
LR Labor room
LSCS Lower segment cesarian section
LUT Lower urinary tract
MAP Mean arterial pressure
MC Menstrual cycle
MESA Microsurgical epididymal sperm aspiration
MIS Mullerian inhibiting substance
MR Menstrual regulation
MRKH Mayer Rokitanksy Kuster Hauser syndrome
MTP Medical termination of pregnancy
MVA Manual vacuum aspiration
NAD No abnormality detected
NS Normal saline
NS Normal size
NST Non-stress test
NTD Neural tube defects
O/E On examination
OC Oral contraceptive
OD Once a day
OPD Outdoor patient department
OT Operation theatre
P/A Per abdominal
P/S Per speculum
P/V Per vaginum
PAC Preanesthetic checkup
PCO Polycystic ovary
PCOS Polycystic ovarian syndrome
PCR Polymerase chain reaction
PESA Percutaneous epididymal sperm aspiration
PGE2 Prostaglandin E2
PID Pelvic inflammatory disease
PIH Pregnancy-induced hypertension
PMB Postmenopausal bleeding
PND Paroxysmal nocturnal dyspnea
POD Pouch of Douglas
POG Period of gestation
POL Progress of labour
POP Progestin only pills
PP Postprandial
PPH Postpartum hemorrhage
PPROM Preterm prelabour rupture of membranes
PPS Postparturm sterilization
PROM Premature rupture of membranes
PTL Preterm labour
PTTK Partial thromboplastin time with kaolin
PT Prothrombin time

PV Per vaginum
PVR Per vaginum/rectum
QOL Quality of life
R & M Routine and microscopic
R & ME Routine and microscopic examination
r/o rule out
R/V Retroverted
RDS Respiratory distress syndrome
RL Ringer lactate
S&E Suction and evacuation
S.AFP Serum alfa feto protein
S/D Systolic/diastolic
S/S Signs and symptoms
SFD Small for dates
SFH Symphysio fundal height
SO Salpingo-oophorectomy
SOS Save our souls (immediately as required)
STD Sexually transmitted disease
SUI Stress urinary incontinence
T/t Treatment
TAH Transabdominal hysterectomy
TCA To come after
TDI Total dose infusion
TDO Transverse diameter of outlet
TESA Testicular sperm aspiration
TESE Testicular sperm extraction
TFT Thyroid function test
Tvl Total vaginal length
TVS Transvaginal sonography
TVT-O Transobturator tension-free tape
UPT Urinary pregnancy test
USG Ultrasonography
UTI Urinary tract infection
VDRL Venereal disease research lab
Vg Vagina
VIA Visual inspection of cervix with acetic acid
VILI Visual inspection of cervix with Lugol's iodine
VVF Vesicovaginal fistula
Vx Vertex
WBC White blood cells
WHO World Health Organization
WNL Within normal limits
wt Weight

Section

1

Obstetrics

- Normal Pregnancy
- Problems in the First-half of Pregnancy
- Problems in the Second-half of Pregnancy
- Delivery of the Fetus and Labour Room Procedures
- Obstetrical Emergencies
- Puerperium
- Contraception and Medical Termination of Pregnancy

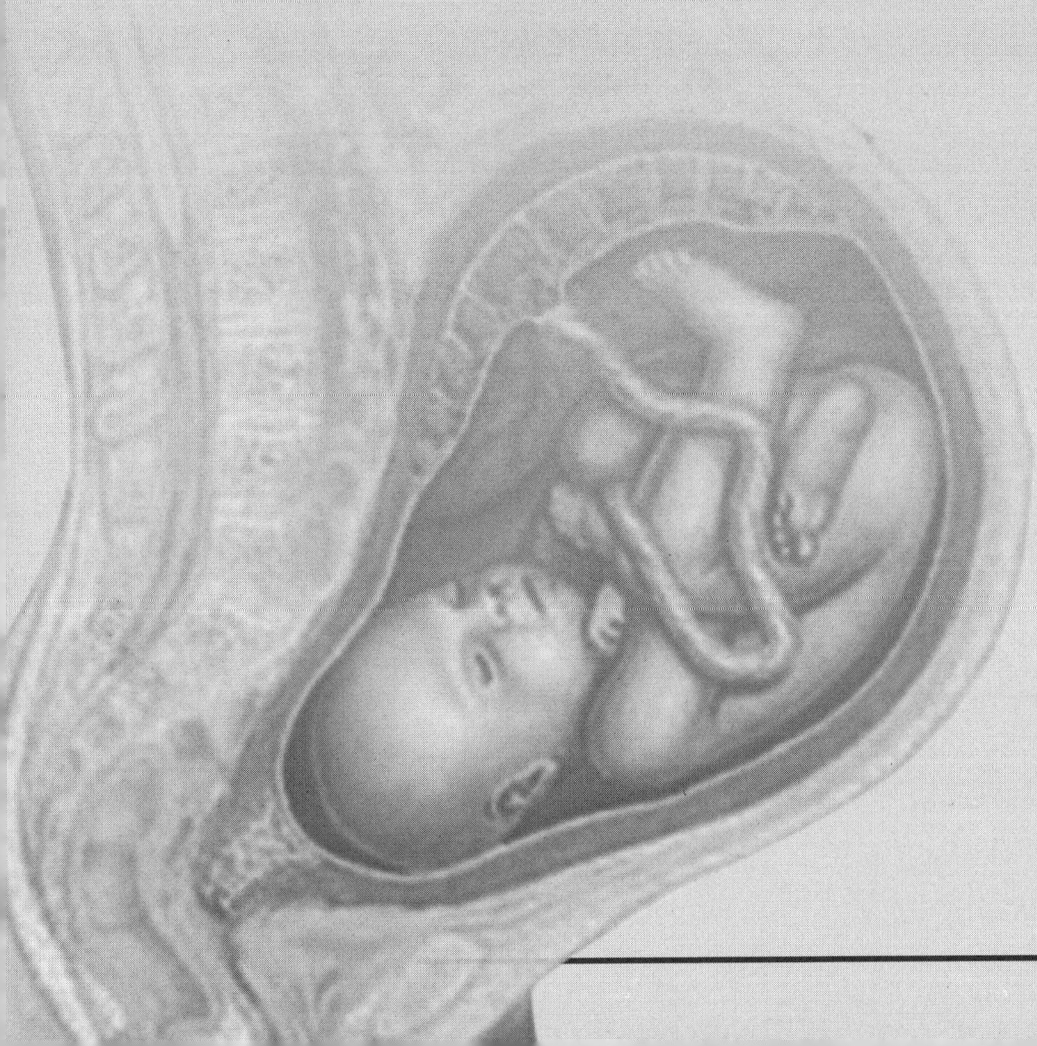

1 Normal Pregnancy

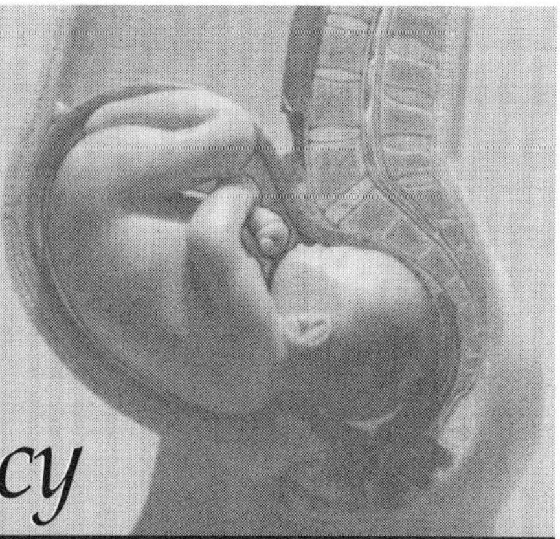

Q1. Why did you ask the woman to report to you for antenatal checkup at regular intervals?

Multiple regular antenatal visits are required so as to:

- Detect and treat existing problems.
- Implement minor but significant interventions to improve the maternal and fetal outcome, e.g. iron/folic acid prophylaxis, tetanus prophylaxis.
- Detect complications arising in pregnancy at an early stage before they become lifethreatening emergencies, e.g. PIH, gestational diabetes. Though PIH is not preventable, early detection and appropriate management can prevent eclampsia.
- Monitor the growth of fetus and detect fetal growth abnormalities at the earliest.

Q2. What is the recommended schedule of visits to the hospital during antenatal care?

The standard visit schedule for antenatal checkup is:

- Every 4 weeks till 28th week.
- Every 2 weeks till 36th week.
- Every week till 40th week.

At peripheral centers with limited resources, only 4 visits are considered

An antenatal card of a pregnant woman whose last menstrual period (LMP) was on 01.01.07 and who delivered on 1.10.07

CASE 1

XYZ 24 years

06.02.07 (1st visit)

Primi ($G_1P_{0+0+0+0}$)

C/o

Amenorrhea 1½ months

Morning sickness

- No history of using any contraception or oral contraceptive pills
- Past medical history–Normal

LMP – 1.01.07

EDD – 8.10.07

POG – 5 weeks + 1 day

O/E

BP	120/80 mmHg
Weight	50 kg
CVS	NAD
Chest	NAD
Pallor	–ve
Breast	NAD, nipples normal
P/s	Cervix blue
P/v	Uterus R/V, soft, bulky, Fx free

Investigations
Urine for pregnancy test
If UPT is positive, then:
- Hb
- Urine (R & M)
- BG (ABO & Rh)
- HB_s Ag
- VDRL
- Voluntary counselling and test for HIV
- NESTROF test

R_x
Tab FA 5 mg 1 OD × 1 month
Tab antiemetic for morning sickness (combination of pyridoxine + dicyclizine), TCA 1 month

06.03.07 (2nd visit)
POG: 9 weeks + 1 day
O/E

Complaints	Nil
BP	120/80 mmHg
Wt	50 kg

Investigation

• Hb	10.8 g dl^{-1}
• Urine (R & M)	NAD
• BG (ABO & Rh)	B+
• VDRL	Non reactive
• Voluntary counselling and test for HIV	Negative
• HB_s Ag	Negative
• NESTROF test	Negative

Adv
Tab FA 5 mg OD × 4 weeks

09.04.07 (3rd visit)
POG: 14 weeks
O/E

BP	120/76 mmHg
Wt	51 kg

P/A uterus just palpable

sufficient for ANC in uncomplicated pregnancies. In the first visit, the patient is registered and the first antenatal check-up is done. The first visit is recommended as soon as the pregnancy is suspected, preferably not later than the first trimester. The second visit should be scheduled between the 4th and 6th month (around 26 weeks). The third visit is planned in the 8th month (around 32 weeks), and the fourth one in the 9th month (36–40 weeks). Additional visits do not improve the maternal or perinatal outcome.

Q3. You have used the code $G_1P_{0+0+0+0}$ for the patient. What does it mean?

The basic elements of obstetric history are gravidity (G), parity (P), and abortions (A). *Gravidity* means number of conceptions including the present one. *Parity* means the number of times the woman has delivered after the age of viability. *Abortion* is the expulsion of products of conception before the age of viability. The numeric subscripts indicate the number of events. Some examples are given below:

i. Primigravida will be presented as $G_1P_0A_0$.
ii. Multigravida with one previous delivery and one abortion will be presented as $G_3P_1A_1$.

The disadvantage of this formula is that it does not give us the number of preterm and term deliveries, or the number of live issues the patient has. This problem is addressed in another scheme of formula in which $G_0P_{0+0+0+0}$, means $G_0P_{term+preterm+abortions+live\ issues}$. Some more examples are given below:

a. $G_2P_{1+0+0+1}$ indicates 1 term delivery with one live issue.
b. $G_3P_{0+1+1+1}$ indicates 1 preterm delivery with one abortion and 1 live issue.
c. $G_3P_{0+1+1+0}$ indicates 1 preterm delivery with one abortion and no live issue.
d. $G_3P_{1+0+1+0}$ indicates 1 term delivery with one abortion and no live issue.

In multiple pregnancies, e.g. second gravida with an earlier twin pregnancy, the parity remains as *one* because she has delivered once irrespective of the number of children delivered. So formula will be $G_2P_{1+0+0+2}$.

Q4. How did you calculate the EDD?

EDD is calculated by adding 9 months and 7 days to LMP. This formula for calculation of the EDD is based on the assumption that the menstrual cycle of the woman was regular before conception and it was a 28–30 days' cycle. 80–90% deliver on EDD ± 7 days, 10% go beyond 42 weeks; these are called prolonged pregnancy or postterm pregnancy. Only 1% of antenatal women deliver on the EDD.

Q5. Why did you examine the breast during antenatal visit?

It is important to examine for the presence of inverted or flat nipples because *inverted nipples* might create a problem in carrying out successful breastfeeding. Examination of breasts during antenatal examination also helps in opportunistic screening for breast malignancies.

Q6. Why did you record the body weight of the woman at each visit?

A pregnant woman's weight should be taken at each visit. The weight taken during the first visit/registration should be treated as the baseline weight. Normally, a woman should gain 9–11 kg during her pregnancy. After the first trimester, a pregnant woman gains around 1–2 kg every month or 0.5 kg per week. Less weight gain raises the suspicion of IUGR, while rapid weight gain may be the earliest sign of pre-eclampsia.

Q7. Why did you prescribe FA routinely during the first 3 months and not thereafter?

Folic acid supplementation is given during first trimester to decrease the risk of neural

Adv

1. Tab FS 100 mg and FA 500 mg — 1 OD
2. Tab calcium — 1000 mg × 1 OD
3. Dietary advise — + 300 Calorie 1 g/kg protein, high milk intake (1L)
4. TCA 4 weeks

07.05.07 (4th visit)

POG: 18 weeks

O/E

BP	110/70 mmHg
Wt	52 kg
Pedal edema	Nil
Pallor	Nil

P/A

- Uterus 18 weeks
- External ballottement present

Investigations

Hb

S.AFP or USG to rule out GCA

R_x

1. CST × 4 weeks
2. Inj TT (0.5 ml i/m) 1st dose
3. TCA 4 weeks

04.06.07 (5th visit)

POG: 22 weeks

Date of quickening: 25.05.07

BP	110/70 mmHg
Wt	53 kg
Pedal edema	Nil
Pallor	Nil

P/A

22 weeks

FPP (Fetal parts palpable)

FHS +

R_x

1. Inj TT (0.5 ml i/m) 2nd dose
2. CST × 4 weeks

02.07.07 (6th visit)
POG: 26 weeks
Fetal movements felt
No c/o of preterm labour/PIH/APH

BP	110/70 mmHg
Weight	54 kg
Pedal edema	Nil

P/A
26 weeks
Fetal parts palpable
FHS +reg
Adv. GCT

R_x
1. CST × 4 weeks

30.07.07 (7th visit)
POG: 30 weeks
No S/s of PTL/PIH
Hb (to be done)

BP	120/80 mmHg
Wt	55 kg
Pallor mild	
Pedal edema	Nil

P/A
30 weeks
Cephalic
FHS + Reg
Liquor adequate

Investigation

GCT	130 mg%

R_x
1. CST × 2 weeks

13.08.07 (8th visit)
POG: 32 weeks
Fetal movements +
No headache, epigastric pain, blurring vision, swelling feet.

tube defects in the fetus. Ideally it should be given periconception, i.e. it should be started at least one month before conception and continued till 3 months of pregnancy. Recommended dosage for this purpose is 400 μg in low risk pregnancy, but as folic acid tablet is available only in the strength of 5 mg, we supplement with 5 mg tablet.

After first trimester folic acid is given along with iron for anemia prophylaxis. For this purpose Government of India recommends 100 mg of elemental iron and 500 micrograms folic acids for 100 days even in pregnancies with normal haemoglobin because iron and folic acid demands are increased in pregnancy and are not met with routine diet.

Q8. What is Glucose challenge test (GCT)? Why did you recommend it at 26th week?

GCT is a screening test for gestational diabetes. In this test, the blood sugar is estimated 1 hour after intake of 50 gm glucose, irrespective of last meal. Normal values are <140 mg%. Abnormal values are to be followed up by glucose tolerance test.

The hormones of pregnancy, like estrogen, progesterone and human placental lactogen induce a state of peripheral insulin resistance resulting in postprandial hyperglycemia and hyperinsulinemia. As gestational diabetes is because of exaggerated physiological changes in glucose metabolism, and these changes are maximally seen after 24 weeks, screening is recommended at 24–28 weeks. If the screening is delayed, the hyper-glycemia persists in third trimester causing adverse fetal effects.

Q9. Why did you ask for complaints like headache, epigastric pain, blurring vision, swelling feet around 32nd week?

These are symptoms of severe PIH.

Q10. Why did you advise AFP and USG at the 18th week?

These are done around 16–18 weeks to screen for congenital anomalies. Maternal serum alpha fetoprotein (AFP) is elevated in neural tube defects (NTD) and reduced in Down's syndrome. In our setup, serum α fetoprotein is not available in the hospital. It costs around Rs. 300–400. USG is more easily available and less costly. Ultrasound scan can rule out gross structural congenital anomalies like anencephaly, spina bifida, and defects of the heart, stomach, kidneys and urinary bladder. If the patient is high-risk for neural tube defect as in cases with previous pregnancy with anencephaly, she should be screened in the first trimester for anencephaly, which can be diagnosed as early as in the 11 weeks.

Q11. When an obstetric USG is done at 16–18 weeks, do you look only for structural defects?

No. Transabdominal USG is also used for fetal biometry (measuring biparietal diameter, femur length, abdominal circumference, etc.) for localizing the placenta (whether it is in upper segment or lower segment), and assessing the adequacy of amniotic fluid.

Q12. Why was the pelvic assessment done at about 38 weeks and not earlier or later?

Fetal head is the best pelvimeter and therefore, it is preferable to wait and watch till 38 weeks by when the *fetal head gets fixed* in the majority of primigravidas with adequate pelvis size, and the pelvic assessment can be deferred till the onset of labour, as in the above case. Earlier assessment is not advised as pelvic examination can stimulate preterm labour.

If the *fetal head is not fixed by 38 weeks*, pelvic contraction is suspected and therefore, a pelvic assessment is done. If there is a contracted pelvis, a cesarean section is done at 38 weeks by when the fetus is mature.

BP 120/78 mmHg
Wt 56 kg
Pallor mild, pedal edema nil

P/A
32 weeks, cephalic
FHS + Reg

R_x
1. CST × 2 weeks

27.08.07 (9th visit)
POG: 34 wks
DFMR adequate
Daily fetal movements adequate
BP 120/78 mmHg
Wt 56.5 kg
Pallor mild, pedal edema Nil

P/A
34 weeks, cephalic
FHS + Reg

Rx
1. CST × 2 weeks

11.09.07 (10th visit)
POG: 36 wks
DFMR adequate
No S/s of PIH
BP 120/80 mmHg
Wt 57 kg
Pallor mild
Pedal edema mild

P/A
36 weeks
Cephalic
FHS + regular
Estimated baby weight 2.4 kg
Liquor adequate

R_x
1. CST × 1 week

18.09.07 (11th visit)
POG: 37 wks

FM adequate	
BP	120/80 mmHg
Wt	58 kg
Rest same	

P/A
Uterus term size
Cephalic fixed
FHS + Regular
Liquor adequate

R_x
1. CST × 1 week

25.09.07 (12th visit)
POG: 38 wks

BP	124/80 mmHg
Wt	60 kg

P/A
Uterus term size
Cephalic fixed 3/5th above
FHS + Regular

R_x
1. CST × 1 week

2.10.07 (13th visit)
POG 39 wks, c/o labour pains

BP	120/90 mmHg
Wt	60 kg

P/A
Uterus term size
Mild uterine contractions present

FHS	+ 140/min, regular
EFW	2.5 kg
Liquor	Adequate

Q13. You have advised hemoglobin estimation on the first visit, and thereafter, at 18 weeks and 30 weeks. Why?

At the least, the Hb level in pregnant women should be estimated at the initial antenatal visit and again at 28 weeks. The initial Hb level serves as a baseline for comparison with the Hb level at 28–30 weeks. At any time in pregnancy, a Hb level below 11 g/dl is considered to be anemia, 7–11 g/dl as moderate anemia, and <7 g/dl as severe anemia.

Q14. What is adequate fetal movements?

Daily fetal movement count is the simplest method of assessment of fetal wellbeing. The criteria for adequacy are subjective and vary. We assume fetal movements to be adequate if there are at least 10 movements per day. Only high-risk patients are instructed to record the daily fetal movement rate (DFMR), starting from 30 weeks till delivery. Others are only asked to ensure that there are at least 10 movements per day.

Q15. What is external ballottement?

External ballottement is a clinical sign of intrauterine pregnancy that is elicited by placing a hand on one side of the uterus and giving a push. When there is fetus in the amniotic fluid sac, the fetus moves away and then bounces back to strike the examiner's hand. This sign is elicitable from 16–20 weeks and is important till we are able to palpate the fetal parts. The sign is absent in molar pregnancy.

Q16. What is quickening?

Quickening is first perception of fetal movements, usually around 16–20 weeks, by the mother. It occurs a little earlier in multigravidas than primigravidas.

Q17. How did you assess the adequacy of liquor?

Liquor is assessed subjectively during abdominal palpation. Objective assessment is done during USG examination by measuring liquor pockets and calculating the *amniotic fluid index*. Maternal abdomen is divided into 4 quadrants by two imaginary lines (vertical midline and transverse line at umbilicus). In each quadrant, the largest liquor pocket is measured and added together. Normal AFI is 5–25 cm.

Q18. How did you calculate the EFW? How did you assess the fetal weight?

There are empirical formulas for calculating the fetal weight, and the most commonly used is Johnson's formula:

EFW = (Symphysiofundal height in cm – S) × 155

S = 13 when presenting part is above 0 station
S = 12 when presenting part is at 0 station
S = 11 when presenting part is below 0 station

Fetal weight is assessed subjectively during abdominal examination. More objective assessment is done using empirical formulas based on BPD, FL and AC measurements made during USG examination. One or other of these formulas are built into the USG machine, which gives direct read-out of the fetal weight.

Q19. What is cervical assessment? How did you perform it?

Cervical assessment is evaluation of the cervix at or near term to assess the likely success of induction of labour in that case.

Cervical assessment is done during P/V examination and the following features of the cervix are noted with fingers: Cervical dilatation in cm, cervical effacement (progressive shortening and thinning of cervix expressed in percentage) cervical consistency (soft, medium, firm), and cervical position

P/V
Cx 50% effaced, 2 cm dilated
BOM +, Vx at -2 station
Pelvic adequate for this baby

Adv
1. Admit LR
2. Watch for **POL**

(posterior, mid, anterior). A 75% cervical effacement means that of the total cervical length of approximately 2.5 cm at term, only 0.6 cm of cervix has remained distinct from the uterus, while the rest of it has 'effaced' and become indistinguishable from the main body of the uterus.

Q20. What is BOM+?

BOM+ means that the bag of membrane is present. During true labour pains, when uterus contracts, intra-amniotic pressure rises and unsupported membranes overlying the presenting part above dilated cervix bulge and become tense. This is known as formation of bag of membranes. This is a sign of onset of labour.

Q21. What is meant by vertex at station-2? What are stations 1, 3, etc.?

Station of vertex (presentation) means relation of the most leading part of fetus in relation with the level of ischial spines. 0 station is at the level of spines. If station is above it is denoted by –ve sign and if below spines, it is denoted by +ve sign. There are two methods of reporting station. In the old method pelvic cavity between pelvic brim and planes of ischial spines and below from ischial spines to outlet is divided in 3 parts each and station is reported to be –3, –2, –1, 0, +1, +2, +3 from above down. Station –3 means, vertex is at pelvic brim, 0 means at the level of ischial spines, +3 means at pelvic outlet. In the new system, in place of 3, cavity above and below 0 station is divided into

Flow Chart 1.1: Evaluation of Nestroft +ve pregnancy

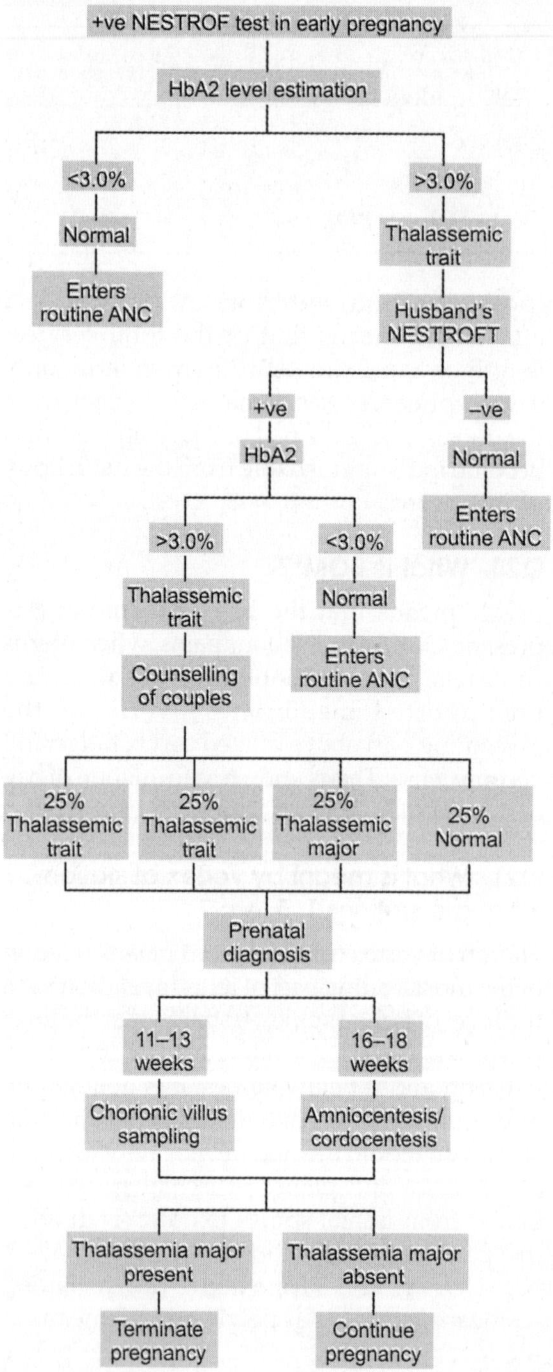

5 parts each. Therefore, the stations are progressively –5, –4, –3, –2, –1, 0, +1, +2, +3, +4, +5 (from inlet to outlet). In this system station corresponds to distance in centimeters. Thus, –5 means 5 cm above 0 station, i.e. ischial spines, +4 means 4 cm below 0 station. This system is more reliable.

Q22. What is NESTROF test?

NESTROF test is *naked eye single tube red cell osmotic fragility test*–a screening test for β thalassemia trait. This test is based on the increased osmotic fragility in thalassemia, which results in greater hemolysis of the RBCs in hypotonic solutions. Hemolysis increases the optical opacity of the solution, which is assessed visually. The test is done in all pregnant women before 18 weeks of pregnancy. The aim is to detect thalassemic fetus before 20 weeks of pregnancy so as to offer termination (Flow Chart 1.1).

Q23. How is NESTROF test done?

Take 2 ml of 0.36% saline and add 0.2 ml of blood. Take another control tube with distilled water and add 0.2 ml of blood (control). Leave tubes undisturbed for 1/2 hr. Keep a white paper/card with a dark line drawn across it behind the tubes. The dark line will be visible across the control tube. If visible through the test tube then result is Negative. If the line is not visible through the test tube: Result is positive.

Q24. What will you do if a pregnant woman tests positive for HIV?

If a pregnant woman tests positive for HIV, she should be counseled about her HIV status, its implications on her health and the risk of its transmission to the fetus. There is 25% risk of perinatal transmission of HIV. She should also be educated on the need for proper antenatal care and the interventions that reduce the risk of transmission to the fetus. The stage of the disease should be assessed clinically. If the woman does not want to continue with the pregnancy, she is offered MTP. If she wants to continue with the pregnancy, the gestational age is confirmed, through USG if required, since an elective cesarean may be required near term. She must also be screened and treated for STDs like Chlamydia, gonorrhoea and hepatitis-B. Her partner must also be tested for HIV and treated if found to be HIV positive.

Antiretroviral therapy (ART) is required for maternal HIV infection if she is in

a. Clinical stage 4,
b. Clinical stage 3 with CD4 <350/mm^3, or
c. Clinical stage 1 or 2 with CD4 <200/mm^3. If the facilities for CD4 test are not available, then ART is given in clinical stage 3 and 4. ART must be started by an HIV specialist after assessing the clinical stage of the disease. Tests like blood glucose, CBC, LFT and KFT are performed before starting ART and at regular intervals thereafter so that its toxicity can be monitored. During the course of treatment, the CD4 cell count and plasma HIV RNA copy number must be ascertained every 3 months to assess the improvement.

In clinical stages when ART is not indicated for maternal HIV infection, ART is given for preventing transmission of HIV infection to the child which usually occurs peripartum. Ideally, the highly active antiretroviral therapy (HAART) should be started at 28–32 weeks, continued intrapartum and stopped postpartum. The infant is given azidothymidine (AZT) for 6 weeks. In India, low cost alternatives are often used, e.g. oral nevirapine single dose of 200 mg given as soon as labour starts (at least 2 hours before delivery). In the infant, nevirapine syrup 2 mg/kg body weight single dose is given within 72 hours of delivery.

Elective LSCS under prophylactic antibiotic cover at 38 weeks is ideal if:

1. The patient is not on HAART,
2. The RNA load is >1000 copies/ml, and
3. The membranes are unruptured.

In ideal situations vaginal delivery is permissible only if the patient is on HAART with a viral load of <1000 copies/ml. Vaginal delivery is considered if the patient so desires or the facilities for LSCS are not adequate as in limited resource settings or if the membranes have ruptured and delivery is imminent. Artificial rupture of membrane, invasive fetal monitoring and fetal sampling, instrumentation and episiotomy are to be avoided in vaginal delivery. Following delivery, the cord should be clamped quickly. The baby should be bathed immediately, taking care to clean its face of maternal fluids.

After delivery, the mother should avoid breastfeeding if good formula feeds are available. If formula feeds are not available or cannot be hygienically administered, as in developing countries, exclusive breastfeeding is recommended for 6 months. Mixed feeds should never be given because it increases the chances of HIV transmission to the neonate: Top feeds always cause some amount of mucosal injury in the intestine of the neonate, which enables the HIV in breast milk to gain entry into the body of the neonate.

2 Problems in the First-half of Pregnancy

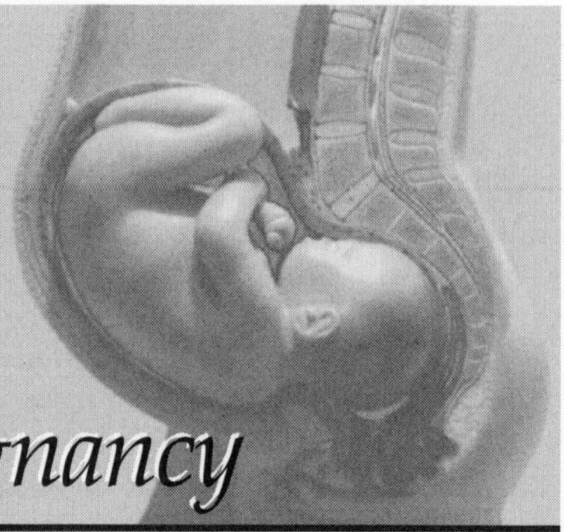

CASE 2A: MISCARRIAGE (Abortion)

A 20-year-old, $G_1P_{0+0+0+0}$
C/o Amenorrhea – 2 months
Bleeding P/V – 1 day
Pain abdomen – 1 day
No h/o passing products of conception
LMP – 2 months back
Previous cycles were of normal duration

O/E
No pallor

Pulse	88/min
BP	110/80 mmHg
Breast	NAD
P/A	NAD
P/S	Cx blue
Bleeding through os +	
P/V	Cx soft and uneffaced Os closed No cervical excitation pain Uterus AV, 8 weeks, mobile, B/L fornix free, nontender
CI	Threatened abortion

Adv
Urgent transvaginal ultrasound
Hb

The problems commonly encountered in the first trimester are bleeding P/V and pain abdomen. Of these, the bleeding P/V is commoner. Another common complaint in the first trimester is nausea and vomiting which, when excessive, it is known as hyperemesis gravidarum.

Sometimes the patient may report to the OPD for the first time with pain abdomen and bleeding P/V. In such cases, it is very important to ask about a history of amenorrr-hoea as she might be pregnant. Pregnancy with *pain abdomen and bleeding P/V* could be due to:

1. Abortion,
2. Molar pregnancy or
3. Ectopic pregnancy.

If bleeding predominates and pain is not much of a problem, then it is either one of the *abortions* or a molar pregnancy. If pain is predominant with spontaneous, irregular infrequent bleeding, then the possibility of *ectopic or tubal gestation* must be considered. The triad can also be due to *delayed period*.

Q1. What are the different types of abortions?

Abortion is the death of the fetus or passage of products of conception (fetus and placenta) before 20 weeks of pregnancy. It is called **early** or **late abortion** depending on whether it occurs *before or after 12 weeks* of gestation. Miscarriage is a preferred term than abortion.

An abortion can be **spontaneous or induced**. Clinically, abortion can be of various degrees. Vaginal bleeding in presence of viable pregnancy is called **threatened abortion** as it signals a danger of spontaneous abortion. If vaginal bleeding or rupture of the membranes is accompanied by cervical dilation, an abortion is unavoidable and is called **inevitable abortion**. If process of expulsion of products of conception has started but not completed, it is **incomplete abortion**. However, if process of expulsion is complete, it is known as **complete abortion**. When there is no embryo in the gestational sac (blighted ovum or anembryonic pregnancy) or an undetected death of embryo/fetus that is not expelled, it is called a **missed abortion**.

Q2. Is bleeding during the first trimester always ominous?

Yes, it is mostly pathological but sometimes bleeding in first trimester can be benign due to **implantation bleeding**, in which slight bleeding occurs around the time of missed period.

Q3. What do you look for in the USG report in a case of abortion?

USG report may show any of the following:

1. Live pregnancy, suggesting threatened abortion as in case 2A(i)
2. Fetal demise, suggesting missed abortion (also called nonviable pregnancy, anembryonic pregnancy, or blighted ovum), as in case 2A(ii).
3. Molar pregnancy.
4. Empty uterine cavity, suggesting ectopic pregnancy, complete abortion or a delayed period. A UPT can exclude the diagnosis of delayed period.

Urine R/M
BG (ABO & Rh)

USG report Case 2A(i)
USG shows live pregnancy
▲ Threatened abortion

Adv.

- Counseling and reassurance.
- Tab folic acid 5 mg 1 OD to continue as in any other pregnancy.
- Micronised progesterone 200 mg BD oral or 200 mg vaginal OD till 14–16 weeks.
- Repeat scan in 2 weeks if bleeding recurs to ensure viability.
- Nuchal thickness at 11 weeks.
- Detailed anomaly scan at 18–20 weeks.

USG Report Case 2A(ii)
The USG shows fetal pole (CRL >6 mm, no cardiac activity, or CRL <6 mm with no change in rescan after 7 days)

▲ Missed abortion or nonviable pregnancy

or

USG report: Gestation sac (diameter >20 mm, no embryonic pole/yolk sac OR diameter is <20 mm with no change in 7 days later).

▲ Anembryonic pregnancy or blighted ovum

Adv.

- Hb, urine (R & M), BG (ABO and Rh), coagulation profile.
- If patient is hemodynamically stable:
  - Vaginal or oral misoprost 400 μg as in medical abortion (patient aborts in 4–6 hours).
- If patient is hemodynamically unstable
  - Suction evacuation.

Q4. Why did you recommend 'transvaginal' ultrasonography? Is not USG commonly done transabdominally?

In first trimester uterus is a pelvic organ and its contents are best assessed by transvaginal sonography. Also transvaginal sonography (TVS) is more effective for diagnosing ectopic pregnancy. If the gestational age is less than 12 weeks, a transvaginal sonography should be done first. Transabdominal USG is done only if transvaginal USG is inconclusive. After 1st trimester, the transabdominal USG is mostly satisfactory, and a transvaginal USG should be done only if transabdominal USG is abnormal or inconclusive.

Q5. How would you diagnostically differentiate incomplete or complete or inevitable abortion?

Clinically in incomplete or complete abortion, there would be h/o passing products of conception and uterus would be smaller than period of amenorrhea. Moreover, ultrasound criteria will be different:

a. In *incomplete abortion,* USG will show heterogeneous tissue (with or without gestation sac) distorting the endometrial midline echo.

b. In *complete abortion,* bleeding is settled and ET is <15 mm.

c. *Inevitable abortion* is a clinical diagnosis and in this case pain is severe, bleeding is excessive. On examination, cervix is ballooned up or os is open and size of uterus is the same as period of gestation.

Q6. How would you manage incomplete/complete/inevitable abortion?

Management of incomplete or inevitable abortion demands evacuation of uterus either medically or surgically depending on the clinical status of patient (*see* answer to missed abortion). In complete abortion, the patient is reassured and a repeat pregnancy test is advised after 2 weeks to ensure that the abortion is indeed complete.

Q7. Will you give Rh immune prophylaxis in Rh -ve mother?

If period of gestation is >12 weeks, then anti-D (250 μg 1/M) should be given. For abortions <12 weeks, 50 μg of anti-D should be given in all cases of induced abortions. For spon-taneous abortions <12 weeks in which no curettage is done (complete abortions), anti- D prophylaxis is controversial as the chances of isoimmunization are very remote, but Indian Society recommends anti-D in all cases of bleeding in first trimester. Anti-D should also be given in all cases of ectopic pregnancies.

Q8. You have mentioned "evacuation of the uterus by surgical means or medical means" as part of the treatment. Can this procedure be called MTP?

No, the term MTP is reserved for medical termination of pregnancy (induced abortion) performed under the MTP Act.

Q1. How did you arrive at the diagnosis of ectopic pregnancy?

Ectopic pregnancy is suspected in a woman in reproductive age group if she has *amenorrhoea* with *spotting* P/V and *pain abdomen*. Clinically cervical excitation pain and tenderness in right fornix favors the diagnosis of ectopic pregnancy.

The diagnosis is confirmed if UPT is positive and a transvaginal USG shows the gestational sac in the adenexa instead of in the uterus. Even a *mixed echogenic mass* in the adenexa is highly suggestive of ectopic pregnancy. A gestational sac may not be seen even in intrauterine pregnancy if serum βHCG level is <2000 IU/L. Therefore, if patient is stable, the serum test is repeated after 48 hours. In normal pregnancy serum βHCG level rises >66% in 48 hours and nearly doubles in 72 hours. If the rise is less and USG is inconclusive, a failing intrauterine pregnancy is also a possibility, and a uterine curettage can be done to detect trophoblastic tissue. However, if the patient is unstable or symptomatic, an urgent laparoscopy or laparotomy is called for.

Q2. What is cervical excitation pain?

Touching or moving the cervix results in pain.

Q3. What are the different common presentations of tubal pregnancy?

Ectopic pregnancy can present as unruptured ectopic, tubal abortion, tubal rupture and chronic ectopic (Table 2.1). In most cases, there is h/o amenorrhea with irregular bleeding, and the UPT is positive. The dictum is that in any woman in reproductive age group with amenorrhea and bleeding P/V ectopic pregnancy should be ruled out.

CASE 2B ECTOPIC PREGNANCY (UNRUPTURED)

25 years $P_{0+0+0+0}$
C/o Amenorrhea – 6 weeks
Severe pain abdomen – 2 days

LMP	6 weeks back
Previous cycles	normal
O/H Infertility	4 years

O/E

Mild Pallor

Pulse	88/min
BP	110/80 mmHg
Chest, CVS	NAD
P/A	NAD
P/S	Cx healthy
P/V	Cervical excitation pain+
	Ut A/V, bulky, soft
	Rt fx extremely tender with 2 × 2 cm palpable mass
	Lt fx free

No bogginess in pouch of Douglas
CI: Ectopic pregnancy

Adv

- UPT +ve
- TVS – No gestation sac in uterus
  ET – thick, 20 mm.

Rt adnexal mass showing sac with small fetal pole but no cardiac activity
Left ovary normal
No free fluid in pouch of douglas.

▲ *Final diagnosis:* Unruptured ectopic gestation

Patient can be considered for medical management.

- *Counseling:* If patient is willing, and prerequisites of medical T/t.
- Take written consent.
- Send βHCG, baseline hemogram with platelets, LFT and KFT, blood group.

- Inj methotrexate 1 mg/kg (Single IM injection).
- Rpt βHCG on D4 and D7 of injection.
- Review weekly clinically + serum hCG until HCG < 5 IU/l.

Q4. Is methotrexate given routinely in ectopic pregnancy?

No, not routinely. The best candidate for methotrexate T/t is a woman with unruptured ectopic pregnancy and:

- Serum βHCG <15,000 IU/L
- Tubal size <4 cm (on ultrasound)
- No fetal cardiac activity
- Compliance for follow-up for several weeks
- Hemodynamic stability.

Lower abdominal pain and bleeding P/V often worsen 2–6 days after methotrexate but it improves quickly. The β-HCG level typically rises on D4 and then starts to fall. Between D4 and D7, if βHCG decrease is <15%, reconsider a second dose and recheck on the 4th day of second injection.

- If βHCG shows a decrease of >15%, then we perform weekly HCG till it is undetectable.

Q5. What are the signs of tubal rupture or treatment failure.

The signs of tubal rupture/treatment failure are:

- Significant worsening of abdominal pain
- Patient is hemodynamically unstable
- Increasing or plateauing levels of beta HCG levels after D7.

Table 2.1: Differentiating features in different types of ectopic presentation

Presentation	*Symptoms*	*Signs*	*Diagnosis basis*	*Treatment*
Unruptured	Asymptomatic or mild symptoms	Hemodynamically stable Tender adenexal mass	USG, serum βHCG	Medical Surgical
Tubal abortion	Mild to moderate pain, spotting/ bleeding	Hemodynamically stable, Mild tenderness, tender illdefined adenexal mass	USG	Surgical Laparoscopy/ laparotomy
Tubal rupture (Ref. case 14B page no. 158)	Severe pain, collapse	Vitals unstable, pt may be in shock P/A: Tenderness, guarding rigidity, Hemoperitoneum+ P/V: very tender, POD fullness Culdocentesis: +(Blood not clotting)	Clinical	Surgical Laparotomy/ laparoscopy
Chronic ectopic	Past h/o acute symptoms-sub-sided, pelvic fullness/pressure, pain during defaecation, dyspareunia, irregular bleeding	Hemodynamically stable, Ill defined pelvic mass in POD, tender	Clinical, USG	Surgical Laparoscopy/ laparotomy

Q1. What is molar pregnancy?

Molar pregnancy also called hydatiform mole is characterized by the presence, in place of a viable fetus, of grape-like structures representing the swollen chorionic villi with trophoblastic hyperplasia. It can be complete (where there is no fetal tissue) or partial (when it contains some fetal tissue).

Q2. How did you arrive at the diagnosis of molar pregnancy?

The clinical features were suggestive of molar pregnancy, which was confirmed through USG. The commonest feature of molar pregnancy is amenorrhea followed by irregular vaginal bleeding. If the uterus is palpable per abdomen, it gives doughy feeling and the fetal parts are not palpable. Internal and external ballottement are not present. If the patient gives history of passing grape-like vesicles per vaginum (a very rare finding), it clinches the diagnosis.

The diagnosis is confirmed mostly through USG. For complete mole, ultrasonogram has a classic picture of "snow storm appearance" created by the multiple small sonolucent areas representing hydropic villi. However, a similar ultrasound picture can also be seen in degenerating fibroid or in placenta of missed abortion. Therefore, a useful adjunct to the diagnosis of molar pregnancy is βHCG levels in serum or urine. βHCG is a specific marker of trophoblastic tissue and correlates precisely with the severity of the disease.

In advanced stages, there is

1. Hyperemesis
2. Anemia
3. Excessive uterine size
4. Theca lutein cyst
5. Pre-eclamsia and
6. Hyperthyroidism.

These features are now rarely encountered due to early diagnosis through the routine use of ultrasound.

CASE 2C MOLAR PREGNANCY

USG report case 2A(iii)

Uterus enlarged

Cavity filled with mixed echogenic mass with small cystic spaces giving snow storm appearance

No fetal tissues seen

B/L ovaries enlarged and multicystic

▲ Hydatidiform Mole or molar pregnancy.

Adv:

- *Hb*
- *Arrange blood*
- Serum βHCG
- X-ray chest PA view
- Suction evacuation in operation theatre

Check curettage after completion

Send tissue for HPE.

Follow up

- Serum βHCG weekly till negative, then monthly for 6 months
- Contraception–minimum till 6 months after βHCG is normal.

Q3. Why was the X-ray chest advised?

The X-ray chest is done to look for trophoblastic metastasis.

Q4. How would you treat this case?

Treatment of molar pregnancy is evacuation of uterus. Suction evacuation is the procedure of choice. There are no fetal tissues/bones, and therefore suction evacuation can be for uterus >12 weeks. Oxytocics are preferably given after the evacuation is complete. However, it may be administered if the patient bleeds before the evacuation is complete. The tissue removed should be sent for histopathology. Sharp curettage should be avoided as there are greater chances of uterine perforation and Asherman's syndrome (uterine synechiae).

Evacuation should be done in operation theatre as there is always risk of severe haemorrhage and respiratory distress due to trophoblastic embolisation.

Medical termination of complete mole and use of strong oxytocics should be avoided because there is a risk of forcing trophoblastic tissue into the circulation causing lung metastasis.

Q5. Why did you advise a 6-month follow-up after the β-HCG levels dropped to normal?

In 20% of patients with complete mole, trophoblastic disease persists and the HCG level does not subside with molar evacuation or levels start rising after it has reached the normal values. The condition is called post-molar gestational trophoblastic neoplasia (GTN). Histologically, it is a form of choreocarcinoma. A greater propensity for malignant transformation of the hydatiform mole is likely if:

1. The maternal age is >40 years,
2. hCG level is >100,000 mIU/ml,
3. There is excessive uterine enlargement, and
4. The theca lutein cyst is >6 cm

It is therefore important to estimate serum levels every week following evacuation till the levels are normal and every month thereafter for 6 months. Clinical examination including per vaginum examination is done every 2–4 weeks to rule out subinvolution of uterus, vaginal and lung metastasis.

Q6. How are complete and partial mole different?

Both are different cytogenetically, pathologically and in their propensity for malignant progression. The only similarity in both is their follow up protocol (βHCG to detect GTN) (Table 2.2).

Q7. When patient should plan her next pregnancy?

Women should be advised not to conceive until the HCG level has been normal for six months. Earlier pregnancy will interfere in follow up of molar pregnancy to detect GTN.

Women who undergo chemotherapy are advised not to conceive for one year after completion of chemotherapy.

Q8. What contraceptive is ideal for them?

The combined oral contraceptive pill are safe to use after HCG levels have reverted to normal. Other forms of hormonal contraception do not appear to be linked to an increased need for treatment.

Table 2.2: Difference between complete mole and partial mole

Complete mole	*Partial mole*
No embryonic or fetal tissue	Embryonic/fetal tissue can be recognized
On microscopy: Diffuse hydropic villi with trophoblastic hyperplasia	Focal trophoblastic hyperplasia
Karyotype is usually diploid (46XX) and is completely paternal	Usually triploid with maternal contribution
May be associated with paraneoplastic or medical sequelae	Resembles spontaneous abortion
Easy to diagnose by signs and symptoms and USG	Mostly retrospective diagnosis or on HPE of conceptus
Persistent trophoblastic disease in 20% of cases	<0.5% of cases

IUCD should not be used as it can lead to prolonged uterine bleeding resulting in interference to evaluate abnormal bleeding.

Q9. Briefly outline the treatment of persistent GTN.

Women with persistent GTN should be treated at a specialist centre with appropriate chemotherapy.

The need for chemotherapy following a complete mole is 15% and 0.5 % after a partial mole (Table 2.2).

Women with evidence of persistent GTN should undergo assessment of their disease followed by chemotherapy. Disease risk is scored according to the FIGO staging for GTN. Women scoring six or less (low risk) receive intramuscular methotrexate on alternate days, followed by six rest days, with each course consisting of four injections.

Women scoring seven or more (high risk) receive combination chemotherapy. The treatment is intravenous etoposide, methotrexate, dactinomycin for two days followed by vincristine and cyclophosphamide (EMA-CO) one week later.

The course is then repeated after one week. Treatment is continued, in all cases, until the HCG level has returned to normal and then for a further 1–3 courses depending on risk category.

CASE 2D RECURRENT ABORTIONS

A 24-year-old $G_4P_0A_3$
c/o 5 weeks amenorrhea
c/o nausea with occasional vomitings

Past obstetrical history

- 3 spontaneous abortions at 6–8 weeks gestation

Pregnancy confirmed by UPT, evacuation done in all
Last abortion 6 months back
Not investigated.
Past medical history: Not significant.
Family history: No family history of mental retardation, congenital defects, still births, recurrent abortions or infertility in first and second degree relatives.

Personal history: No history of any addictions.

O/E

Average built
Vitals—Normal, Thyroid—Not enlarged
Chest/ CVS—NAD, P/A—NAD
P/S—Cervix bluish, P/V—Cervix soft,
Os closed, uterus anteverted, bulky soft, bilateral fornices free
Clinical diagnosis: 24 years old $G_4P_0A_3$ with 5 weeks pregnancy with h/o recurrent early abortions.

Adv:

- UPT
- *USG:* TVS for confirmation of intra-uterine pregnancy, gestational age and viability
- *Routine investigations as in all pregnancies:* Hb, Blood group, VDRL and HIV both partners, Thalassemia Screen, Urine R/M
- *Special investigations for recurrent abortions:* Blood sugars fasting and PP, Thyroid profile, Lupus anticoagulant, anticardio-lipin antibodies (IgG & IgM)

Q1. Following how many abortions is a patient diagnosed as a case of recurrent abortions?

Recurrent abortion is traditionally defined as three or more consecutive abortions occurring before 20 weeks post-menstruation. Early abortions are those in which pregnancy losses occur before 12 weeks.

Q2. What are the causes we look for in a case of recurrent early abortions?

A woman with recurrent first trimester losses needs to be investigated for possible causes:

- *Chromosomal anomalies:* Karyotyping of both partners
- *Endocrinological disorders:* Diabetes and thyroid screening
- *Immunological disorders:* Antiphospholipid antibodies (LA & ACA).
- Luteal phase defects (LPD).

Q3. Should such a case be investigated for TORCH infections?

There is no association between recurrent abortions and infections except for bacterial vaginosis which can cause second trimester losses. Infections *can* cause isolated spontaneous abortions but not recurrent losses. Therefore TORCH investigation is not warranted in a case of recurrent abortions.

Q4. Why do we investigate for LA and ACA?

Up to 15% of women with recurrent pregnancy losses have autoimmune factors. The best established autoimmune disorder associated with recurrent abortions is the *antiphospholipid antibody syndrome* (APS). Antiphospholipid antibodies are diagnosed by testing for lupus anticoagulant (LA) and anticardiolipin antibodies (ACA) medium or high titres. For diagnosis, test results should be positive on two occasions 6 weeks apart. Women with recurrent abortions in whom other causes have been ruled out should be investigated for APS, since specific therapy can improve pregnancy outcome in this condition.

Q5. Do you investigate for APS only in cases of recurrent abortions?

No, we also investigate for APS even if there is a single unexplained fetal deaths at or beyond 10th week. It is also done in severe pre-eclampsia or placental insufficiency-conditions that necessitate delivery before 34th week of pregnancy. Other indications are unexplained vascular thrombosis.

Q6. Why was vaginal progesterone administered to the patient?

Progesterone supplementation is usually given empirically in cases of unexplained abortions till 14th week. It is useful in cases of established LPD. However, its role is not well proven in unexplained abortions.

- Peripheral blood karyotyping of both partners

Treatment: Assurance and tender loving care.

- Avoid heavy work
- Folic acid 5 mg OD
- Vaginal progesterone 200 mg twice a day
- If LA/ACA positive: Low dose aspirin 75 mg OD
- Heparin/low molecular weight heparin
- Treatment continued till term.

Q7. What is the prognosis if no cause is found on investigations?

A significant proportion of cases of recurrent abortion remain unexplained, despite detailed investigation. These women can be reassured that the prognosis for a successful future pregnancy with supportive care alone is in the region of 75%.

CASE 2E HYPEREMESIS GRAVIDARUM

A 24-year-old $G_2P_1L_1A_0$ with amenorrhea 7 weeks
c/o nausea and vomiting × 1 week
Not able to take anything orally for 2 days
No H/o any pain abdomen, bleeding p/v
No H/o fever, urinary complaints

Obst history
Ist pregnancy: FTNVD 2 years, baby is alive and healthy
h/o severe vomiting in first trimester, required hospital admission twice

Past history: No h/o any chronic illness, GI or renal disease, diabetes, etc.

O/E
Patient conscious, oriented, dehydrated
Pallor- nil
P: 100/min, BP: 100/70 mmHg
P/A: NAD, P/S: Cervix blue, NAD
P/V: Cervix soft, os closed, Uterus AV, 8 weeks, mobile, B/L fornices free

Clinical diagnosis: $G_2P_1L_1A_0$ with 7 weeks pregnancy with Hyperemesis Gravidarum
Adv: Admit in Hospital

Investigations
- Blood sugar
- Serum electrolytes
- LFT, KFT
- Thyroid function test
- Urine routine examination including ketones
- Urine culture
- USG to r/o multiple gestation, molar pregnancy

R_x: Nil orally
Reassure patient regarding benign nature of the condition
I/V fluids ringer lactate/DNS

Q1. How is hyperemesis gravidarum different from the vomiting that is common early in pregnancy?

Nausea and vomiting is common during first trimester of pregnancy, affecting 70–80% of women. Usually it is mild and commonly known as morning sickness. When it is severe affecting general health of the woman and requiring hospitalization, it is known as hyperemesis gravidarum. Diagnosis is made after excluding other causes of vomiting like gastrointestinal conditions, genitourinary, metabolic, febrile causes and jaundice, etc.

Q2. When would you admit a case of hyperemesis gravidarum to the hospital?

The indications for admission to hospital are:
1. Persistent vomiting when woman is not able to take anything orally including fluids,
2. Acute starvation as evidenced by ketonuria, and
3. Vomiting causing weight loss.

Q3. How would you manage a simple case of morning sickness in pregnancy?

The general measures are:
1. Avoiding spicy or fatty food,
2. Take small frequent meals rich in carbohydrates and proteins,
3. Eating bland or dry food, e.g. biscuits in the morning before arising, and
4. Taking rest and avoiding stress.

Drug therapy comprises vitamin B_6 10–25 mg 3–4 times per day. Doxylamine 12.5 mg 3–4 times per day is added if required. In majority of the cases, the symptoms improve with these measures and generally subside after first trimester.

Q4. What treatment is given if symptoms not controlled with above measures?

Step wise treatment of nausea and vomiting in pregnancy is given as follows.

Flow Chart 2.1

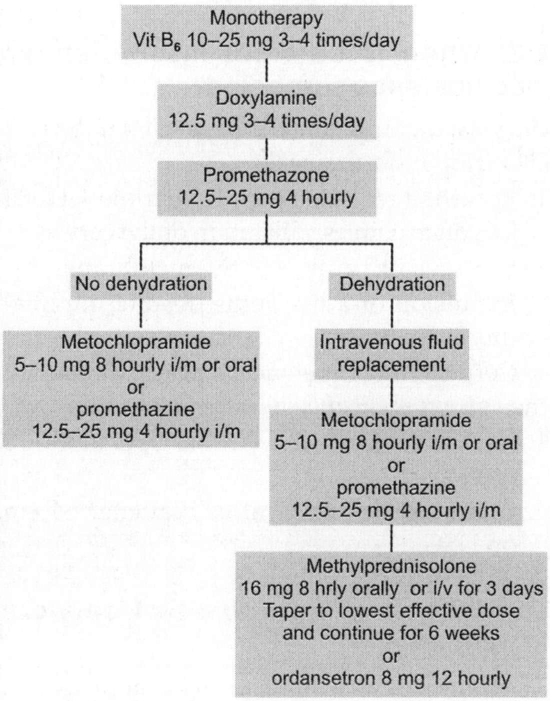

Correction of electrolyte imbalance

Give dextrose if ketonuria present

Add multivitamin infusion in IV fluids

Inj Metoclopramide 5–10 mg IV 8 hourly or Inj Promethazine 12.5–25 mg 4 hourly

Intake/output monitoring, vital monitoring

Urinary ketones and serum electrolytes check 4–6 hourly till corrected

Once vomiting are controlled gradually introduce oral fluids followed by solids

Switch over to oral medication.

CASE 2F CERVICAL INSUFFICIENCY/ INCOMPETENCE

$G_4P_{0+2+1+0}$ with 8 weeks amenorrhea reported for antenatal checkup UPT positive 2 weeks back

Obst history

Ist: Preterm vaginal delivery of live fetus at 24 weeks, H/o PPROM present. Baby died few hours after delivery 4 years back

2nd: Preterm vaginal delivery of live fetus at 29 weeks, short labour of 2 hours, baby remained in nursery for 1 week, died due to Respiratory distress syndrome.

3 years back

3rd: Spontaneous abortion at 18 weeks, painless expulsion of fetus, no congenital anomaly. 1 year back.

No other significant history.

O/E

General examination: Normal

P: 90/min, BP: 120/80 mmHg

Chest/CVS: NAD

P/A: NAD

P/S: Cervix bluish, vagina healthy

P/V: Cervix soft, 2.5 cm long, os closed

Uterus anteverted, 8 weeks, soft

B/L fornices free

Clinical diagnosis

$G_4P_{0+2+1+0}$ with 8 weeks pregnancy with bad obstetric history with cervical insufficiency.

Adv

USG: TVS for confirmation of intrauterine pregnancy, gestational age and viability.

Hb, blood group, VDRL and HIV, thalassemia screen, GCT, TSH, urine R/M, urine c/s

Repeat USG at 13–14 weeks to rule out congenital anomalies

Plan: Cervical cerclage at 14 weeks.

Q1. What is cervical incompetence?

Cervical incompetence is characterised by painless dilatation of the cervix in the second or early third trimester, followed by premature rupture of the membranes and preterm delivery or abortion.

Q2. When is cervical insufficiency/ incompetence suspected?

Cervical incompetence is suspected if the *past obstetrical history* reveals:

1. Recurrent second or early third trimester fetal loss after painless dilatation of the cervix,
2. Prolapse or rupture of the membranes, or
3. Expulsion of a live fetus despite minimal uterine activity.

Cervical incompetence is also suspected if the *current pregnancy* is associated with:

1. Cervical length <2.5 cm on USG at 16–18 weeks, or
2. Open internal cervical os diameter >1 cm on USG.

Q3. What are the causes of cervical incompetence?

The common causes of cervical incompence are:

- Surgical trauma to the cervix
- Conization
- Loop electrosurgical excision procedures
- Overdilatation of cervix during MTP
- Obstetric lacerations
- Congenital mullerian anomalies
- *In utero* exposure to DES
- Deficiencies in cervical collagen and elastin (idiopathic).

Q4. Can cervical incompetence be diagnosed in the non-pregnant state?

In a suggestive history, the following tests can be performed in the nonpregnant state for diagnosing incompetence, but their usefulness is doubtful.

- Ease of passage of size 8 Hegar's dilator.
- *Foley's traction test:* Foley catheter with a 1 ml balloon is inserted beyond the internal os. The balloon is inflated to 1 ml and traction is applied onto the Foley catheter. According to the degree of traction that is required to pull the Foley out of the cervix the diagnosis of competent or incompetent cervix can be made.
- Hysterosalpingogram (done in pre-menstrual phase) demonstrating cervical funneling.

Q5. What is the treatment of cervical incompetence?

Treatment is surgical with cervical cerclage procedure consisting of reinforcement of weak cervix by some type of purse-string suture. Cervical cerclage procedure can be performed as prophylactic procedure or as emergency/urgent cerclage. Based on timing, one may differentiate between

- Prophylactic cerclage prior to conception,
- Prophylactic cerclage in pregnancy,
- Urgent cerclage after shortening of the cervix, and
- Emergency cerclage after exposure of the membranes.

Most commonly performed procedure is prophylactic cerclage performed at 14–16 weeks in women with classical history suggestive of cervical incompetence. In women with doubtful history as an alternative to prophylactic cerclage a policy of serial cervical length measurements can be adopted. Urgent or emergency cerclage is performed after cervical shortening or dilatation with or without bulging of the membranes.

Procedure

McDonald

- Simple, vaginal
- No. 2 Silk suture
- *Level of stitch:* Encircle the body of cervix just below internal os, at the highest level of portio vaginalis.

Shirodker

- Complicated, vaginal
- 5 mm mersilene tape
- *Level of stitch:* Submucosally around cerix at the level higher than McDonald at the level of internal os.

Q6. When should the prophylactic cerclage procedure be done?

The preferred timing of cerclage is at 14–16 weeks of gestation. In case of previous mishaps procedure is due at least 2–4 weeks before the time of previous abortion. Cerclage procedure is usually done after first trimester as most of the abnormal fetuses abort in first trimester and anomalies can be detected on USG before the procedure in second trimester. Moreover by this gestation placenta has taken over the function of corpus luteum so that there are less chances of abortion because of anesthetic or surgical interference.

Q7. When do you perform transabdominal cerclage procedure?

Transabdominal cerclage has been advocated as a treatment for second trimester abortion and the prevention of early preterm labour in selected women with previous failed transvaginal cerclage and/or a very short and scarred cervix when transvaginal procedure is not technically possible.

Q8. When should the cerclage suture be removed?

The suture should be removed, at the completion of 37 weeks, when there is rupture of membranes, or whenever patient goes in labour and contractions start–whichever is the earliest.

Q9. Is cerclage perfectly safe?

No. It has complications like:

1. Rupture of membranes,
2. Chorioamnionitis,
3. Suture displacement, and
4. Premature uterine contractions.

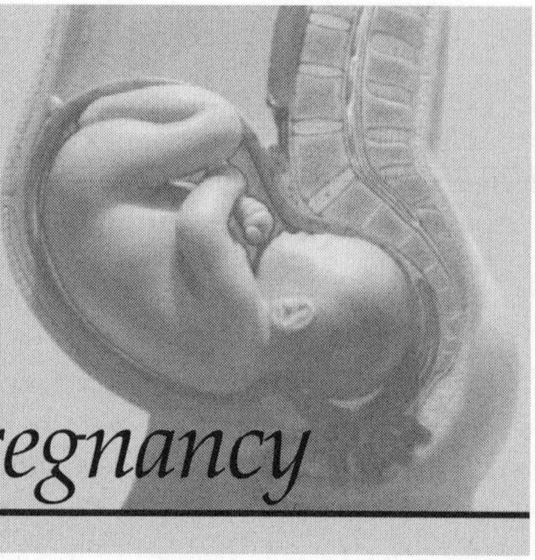

3 Problems in the Second-half of Pregnancy

CASE 3A GESTATIONAL DIABETES

A 30-year-old $G_2P_1L_0$ with 7 months amenorrhea reported to OPD with high blood sugars (Fasting 140 mg/dL).

Pregnancy unsupervised except for 1 visit 1 month back when she was advised investigations.

HOPP: Present pregnancy was diagnosed by clinical symptoms and no examination or tests were done in early pregnancy.

Had only one ANC in the past

Received 1 TT

Took iron and calcium supplements irregularly for 1 month

Obst history: $G_2P_1L_0$

Ist: Spontaneous conception, unsupervised pregnancy, delivery at home with difficulty in second stage, fresh stillbirth of a big baby: 1 year back. No investigations during or after last delivery.

Family history: Mother is diabetic

Examination: Obese

Height: 150 cm, *Weight:* 80 kg

Pallor: Mild

BP: 120/80 mmHg

Diabetes during pregnancy can be pregestational diabetes (i.e. diabetes diagnosed before pregnancy) or gestational diabetes, which is defined as carbohydrate intolerance of variable severity with its onset (or diagnosis) during pregnancy.

Pregestational diabetes is staged using White classification which emphasizes that end organ derangements, especially those involving the eyes, kidneys and heart, have significant effects on pregnancy outcome. The longer the durations of diabetes, the more advanced the staging.

Gestational diabetes occurs because placental hormones tend to increase the blood glucose concentration. It is generally asymptomatic and is usually identified by screening of pregnant women. Often, a pregnant woman develops hyperglycemia later in pregnancy. Therefore, screening test for gestational diabetes is done at 24–28 weeks. Gestational diabetes is categorized as class A1 that is controllable on diet and class A2 that is not controllable on diet and requires insulin therapy. Women with gestational diabetes who maintain fasting glucose levels <95 mg/dl and 2 hour postprandial levels ≤120 mg/dl on diet therapy and exercise (Class A1) do not require any insulin therapy. Such women are at minimum risk for fetal/neonatal complications and weekly monitoring for glucose levels is sufficient. Class A2 women are at high risk for all the complications as seen in pregnancies with pregestational diabetes.

Q1. Why do you diagnose this case as gestational diabetes? How can we be sure that this patient was not diabetic before she conceived?

The presence of gestational diabetes does not exclude the possibility of unrecognized pregestational diabetes. In this case, diabetes is diagnosed for the first time during this pregnancy and therefore, it is labeled as gestational diabetes. But, since the fasting blood glucose is 140 mg/dl, there is a strong possibility of unrecognized preexisting diabetes. Family history, past obstetric history and obesity are also suggestive.

Q2. Do you always screen with oral GCT in pregnancy? Why is GCT not done in the present case?

No, we do not always screen with GCT (glucose challenge test) in pregnancy. When the suspicion of undiagnosed pregestational diabetes is high as in this case, a random or fasting plasma glucose is obtained to confirm diabetes. A fasting glucose level >125 mg/dl or a random sample ≥ 200 mg/dl will confirm diabetes and there is no use of glucose challenge–rather it can be harmful. If these values are normal then GCT is done.

The screening test for gestational diabetes is the glucose challenge test (GCT) with 50 gm oral glucose. GCT is only a screening test and is considered abnormal if the plasma glucose is ≥140 mg/dl. If plasma glucose is ≥ 200 mg/dL following GCT, then fasting plasma glucose is measured and diabetes diagnosed if it is >125 mg/dl. If the value is less, then the complete oral GTT (glucose tolerance test), which is a diagnostic test, is done.

Chest/CVS: NAD
P/A: Uterus 28 weeks, single fetus, longitudinal lie with cephalic presentation.
FHS: 140/min, regular
Uterus relaxed, liquor adequate
P/S: No discharge

Diagnosis: $G_2P_1L_0$ with 28 weeks pregnancy with gestational diabetes

Investigations
Hb, blood group, VDRL, urine R/M
24 hours urine protein, urine C/S, KFT, Fundus
Obstetrics USG with detailed anomaly scan

Management
Diabetic diet: 1800 cal/day
Exercise
Blood sugar profile after 7 days

Q3. How is oral GTT performed in pregnancy?

GTT is performed after an overnight fast of 8–14 hours after 3 days of unrestricted carbohydrate intake. Venous plasma glucose levels are measured fasting 1, 2 and 3 hours after ingestion of 100 gm of glucose with water. The diagnosis of GDM is made when two or more values meet or exceed the cut off thresholds. Two sets of values are recommended by different groups, nowadays trend is towards using lower cut off values (Table 3.1).

Table 3.1: ACOG 2001 criteria for diagnosis of gestational diabetes using 100 gm GTT (Plasm values in mg/dl)

Status	*Carpenter and coustan*	*National diabetic group*
Fasting	95	105
1 hr	180	190
2 hr	155	165
3 hr	140	145

Q4. Why have you done a urine C/s in this case although the patient is not symptomatic of UTI?

The urine C/s is done to diagnose the complications of diabetes like UTI which can be asymptomatic. For the same reason, tests like the KFT and fundus examination are done for early diagnosis of nephropathy and retinopathy that occur in long-standing unrecognized diabetes. During pregnancy, nephropathy is suggested by 500 mg or more proteinuria per 24 hours measured before 20 weeks of pregnancy.

Q5. Are there any risks to pregnancy if a diabetic woman with poor glycemic control conceives?

Yes, during embryogenensis, from conception through the first 8 weeks of gestation, infants born to women with diabetes have a marked increased risk of major congenital anomalies. The risk increases when poor glycemic control is present during embryogenensis. The risk increases up to 22–25% and correlates with initial glycosylated hemoglobin levels and initial mean fasting plasma glucose level. The risk of congenital malformations in diabetic pregnancy can be reduced to the same level as for nondiabetic population by achieving euglycemic control (glycosylated hemoglobin A_{1C} levels <7%) *before* pregnancy.

The other pregnancy risks associated with poor glycemic control are those of spontaneous abortion, unexplained fetal demise, macrosomia, hydramnios and preterm birth. After birth, the neonate often suffers from respiratory distress, hypoglycemia, hypocalcemia, hyperbilirubinemia and cardiac hypertrophy.

Stillbirths without any identiable cause (unexplained fetal demise) are a phenomenon that is peculiar to pregnancies complicated by diabetes. They are called unexplained because no known factors such as placental insufficiency, abruption, fetal growth restriction, oligohydramnios, are apparent. These infants are typically large for age and die before labour usually after 34 weeks of gestation. The incidence of unexplained stillbirths is approximately 1%.

Q6. What special tests are done in diabetic pregnancy other than those in routine ANC?

Special monitoring during pregnancy with diabetes:

- Early establishment of reliable criteria for pregnancy dating by doing USG as early as pregnancy is diagnosed, preferably transvaginal scan in first trimester
- Maternal Serum α feto-protein at 16–20 weeks to diagnose congenital defects (CNS)
- Detailed anatomy scan at 18–22 weeks including fetal echocardiography.

Q7. Why are you not doing glycosylated hemoglobin in this case?

Glycosylated hemoglobin HbA_{1c} levels indicate glycemic control during preceding 4–8 weeks. This is an important test if diabetic woman is seen in first trimester, so that its value can indicate glycemic control around conception and therefore, the risk of congenital malformations. At 28 weeks, it does not have any role, as in the present case.

Q8. How do you monitor for fetal well being in such a case?

Antepartum testing is recommended in all women with pregestational diabetes or insulin requiring GDM at 32–34 weeks of pregnancy or earlier if there are other medical complications or poor glycemic control.

In cases of gestational diabetes controlled on diet (Class A1), antepartum monitoring is done at 38–40 weeks.

Monitoring is done by:
- Daily fetal movement record
- NST weekly
- BPS biweekly

If glycemic control is poor then monitoring frequency is increased.

Q9. Are there maternal complications in pregnancy with diabetes?

Yes, these include infections like candidal infections and UTI, pre-eclampsia and ketoacidosis. The fetal macrosomia associated with diabetis may cause cephalo-pelvic disproportion or shoulder dystocia. There is also an increased risk of postpartum haemorrhage during the third stage of labour.

Q10. How many USG examinations need to be done in a case of pregnancy with diabetes?

In a pregestational diabetic woman, antenatal care should start as soon as she conceives and she will require multiple USGs:

1. First trimester USG (preferably TVS) for exact dating of pregnancy. This is important to avoid unnecessary premature delivery when elective delivery is planned at term.
2. 2nd trimester scan at 18–20 weeks (Detailed anatomical scan also known as level II scan) for congenital malformations.
3. Repeated scans in third trimester after 30–32 weeks to check fetal growth and biophysical scoring (generally every 2 weeks).

Q11. How do you manage diabetes in pregnancy?

Management of diabetes during pregnancy involves dietary therapy, exercise, insulin therapy and fetal surveillance. Women with *pregestational diabetes*, if not on insulin therapy, should be promptly switched to insulin as soon as pregnancy is diagnosed. Their insulin should be titrated to achieve euglycemia. These patients often require multiple injections daily adjusted according to glucose levels. Medical management *of gestational diabetes* begins with a trial of diabetic diet therapy and daily exercise. In women with persistent hyperglycemia despite this, insulin therapy is started as shown in Table 3.2. The initial dose should be based on current gestatinal age and body weight.

Ideally, the monitoring of glycemic control involves seven samples for glucose levels, at fasting, prelunch and predinner, postmeal samples (2 hours after breakfast, lunch and dinner), and midnight sample between 2–6 am. Ideally in a woman on insulin therapy, daily self monitoring of glucose levels should be done at home by glucometer and weekly monitoring of plasma sugar levels in the lab. In cases of gestational diabetes not on insulin, weekly monitoring is enough. The goal of diabetic therapy is to maintain the fasting glucose at 60–95 mg/dl, 1 hour postprandial glucose at <140 mg/dl, 2 hour postprandial glucose at <120 mg/dl, and the night levels (2–6 am) at 60–90 mg/dl.

For pregestational diabetes and gestational diabetics on insulin, the delivery is done at 38

Table 3.2: General guidelines for starting doses of insulin therapy

Trimester	*Total units of insulin*	*Twice daily*	*Split dose*
1st	0.6–0.7 units/kg	AM: 2/3 of total	Short acting: 2/3 of AM
2nd	0.7–0.8 units/kg		Intermediate acting: 1/3 of AM
3rd	0.8–0.9 units/kg	PM: 1/3 of total	Short acting: 1/2 of PM
			Intermediate acting: 1/2 of PM

weeks. For gestational diabetes on diet control, it is conducted at the usual 40 weeks. But if there are medical or obstetrical complications or any fetal compromise, an elective delivery/cesarean section is conducted before 38 weeks.

In diabetic women on insulin, insulin requirement decrease after delivery. After 24–48 hours, once woman is taking full diet, she is started on half the dose of insulin required before and then dose adjusted with blood sugar levels. Women with gestational diabetes should be tested between 6 and 12 weeks post-delivery for diabetes by oral GTT with 75 gm glucose to diagnose diabetes. If normal she should be tested annually thereafter. Women with h/o GDM will have a >50% chance of developing diabetes within 10–20 years.

At discharge, the mother is advised to continue diabetic diet, exercise daily, and to achieve and maintain the ideal body weight. If her 6 weeks postpartum GTT is normal, she can opt for any contraceptive like the progestogen-only pills, low dose combined pills (after 6 months if breastfeeding), IUCD or the barrier contraceptives.

Q12. Can the mother be given insulin or oral hypoglycemic drugs during lactation?

Insulin, yes, but oral hypoglycemics are contraindicated during lactation.

Q1. What was the cause of breathlessness in this patient?

The patient has severe anaemia and pulmonary edema (evidenced by the basal crepitations). Both cause breathlessness. Other pregnancy-related causes of breathlessness are pre-eclampsia and concealed abruptio placentae, both of which are associated with pulmonary edema. This can also be due to associated cardiac disease.

Q2. Is cardiac failure common in pregnancy? If so, why?

Pregnancy predisposes to cardiac failure because of profound hemodynamic changes (increase in blood volume and increase in cardiac output). These changes start in the first trimester and increase till third trimester. Cardiac disease or severe anemia, when present, imposes an additional stress that the heart is not able to cope up with, resulting in cardiac decompensation. In majority of the cases, the cardiac failure occurs peripartum when there are further hemodynamic burdens during uterine contractions and delivery of fetus and placenta.

Q3. Is anemia common in pregnancy? If so, why?

Pregnancy increases the demand of nutrients, especially iron. About 850 mg of extra iron is required during pregnancy. Diet alone cannot meet this extra requirement and therefore iron supplementation is necessary in pregnancy. Malnutrition and worm infestation, which are common in our country, and multiple pregnancies at short intervals aggravate nutritional deficiency. This patient is unsupervised and has never taken iron and folic acid supplementation during pregnancy.

There is another cause for anemia that is not related to pregnancy: Hookworm is endemic (prevalence of 20% or more) in our country and deworming therapy should be

CASE 3B SEVERE ANEMIA WITH CARDIAC FAILURE IN PREGNANCY

A 30-year-old $G_4P_3L_3$
C/o Amenorrhea 32 weeks
C/o acute breathlessness for 2 hours
No h/o labour pains or leaking P/V or bleeding P/V
Perceiving fetal movements adequately

HOPP: H/o dyspnoea on exertion for one month. No h/o orthopnoea/PND.
H/o palpitations, lethargy for similar duration
No h/o chest pain, cyanotic or syncopal attacks,
Unbooked unsupervised pregnancy.
Pregnancy diagnosed by fetal movements at 4 months
Only two visits in dispensary for TT immunization
No investigations done and not taking any haematinics

Obst history: $G_4P_3L_3$
All full term babies, at an interval of 1 to 2 years, A&H
No complications in antepartum or postpartum period
Last child birth: 2 years

Menstrual history: Conceived in lactational period
No contraception used
Socioeconomic status of patient is poor

O/E: Patient breathless, RR- 20/minute
Pallor severe, prominent neck veins, JVP-increased
Pulse: 100/min, reg
BP: 110/70 mmHg
Pedal edema ++
Chest-basal crepitations +
CVS: Ejection systolic murmur +

P/A: Liver palpable 1 finger below costal margin and tender with positive hepatojugular reflex
Uterus enlarged, Fundal height 32 weeks
Single fetus, cephalic, FHS: 130/min, regular
Uterus relaxed, non tender, not tense
Abdominal wall edema +
L/E: No Bleeding P/V, vulvar edema +

Diagnosis: $G_4P_3L_3$ with 32 weeks pregnancy with severe anemia with cardiac failure with anasarca

Management:
Admit in Obstetric emergency
Bed rest in propped up position
Oxygen by mask
Give injection lasix 20 mg i/v stat
Strict intake/output charting
Arrange for packed red cells transfusion

Investigations:
Complete hemogram with platelet count with RBC indices with P/S for type of anemia and MP
LFT with serum proteins
KFT
ECG and X-ray chest
Urine R/M
Stool test for ova/cyst, occult blood
Obstetric USG for fetal growth (only once maternal condition is stable and she has recovered from cardiac failure)

Arrange and transfuse two units red cell concentrates under lasix cover (slow transfusion under constant supervision)

Once patient comes out of cardiac failure and investigations confirm iron deficiency anemia she will be given injectable iron therapy and oral folic acid.

given to every anemic mother due to iron deficiency. Any one of the following anthelminthic treatments can be prescribed: Albendazole 400 mg oral once or mebendazole 500 mg once or 100 mg two times per day for 3 days OR levamisole 2.5 mg/kg body weight oral once daily for 3 days or pyrantel 10 mg/kg body weight once daily for 3 days.

Q4. Why do you call this a case of severe anemia?

According to WHO, hemoglobin level below 11 gm/dl in pregnant woman constitutes anemia and Hb below 7 gm/dl is severe anemia. ICMR uses four categories of anemia:

Category	*Anemia severity*	*Hemoglobin level (g/dl)*
1	Mild	10.0–10.9
2	Moderate	7.0–10.0
3	Severe	<7.0
4	Very severe (decompensated)	<4.0

Clinically her pallor suggested Hb <7 g% and anemia was complicated by cardiac failure, therefore it was diagnosed as severe anemia.

Q5. Why was this patient advised blood transfusion instead of iron therapy?

This patient was advised blood transfusion because her anemia was severe and complicated by cardiac failure.

Q6. What factors make you decide whether patient needs blood transfusion or oral or parenteral iron?

Oral iron therapy	Pregnancy <30 weeks, since it is by far the safest mode of administration of iron, and is as effective as parenteral iron therapy. With 10 weeks more to delivery, there is enough

	time to switch the patient to parenteral iron in case of intertolerance to oral iron or if the patient is noncompliant
Parenteral iron (IM or IV)	Pregnancy 30–36 weeks, since with the delivery only a few weeks away, there is little time to take chances with the oral iron therapy. It is also given at <30 weeks if the patient is intolerant to oral iron or is noncompliant
Blood transfusion	Pregnancy >36 weeks, since it is the quickest way to increase Hb. It is also given irrespective of gestation if the patient develops cardiac failure due to severe anemia.

Q7. How much blood should be transfused in this patient?

Packed cell transfusion should be done. Each unit of RBCs is supposed to increase haemoglobin by 1 to 1.5 gm/dl and haematocrit by 3 to 5%. RBCs should be transfused slowly under diuretic cover in decompensated patient. Once the patient is out of acute stage and investigations reveal it to be iron deficiency anemia, she is parenterally administered the total required dose of iron calculated by the formula:

Total iron requirement in mg =

$$2.21 \times \text{Weight of patient in kg} \times (\text{normal Hb} - \text{patient's Hb in gm/dl}) + 1000 \text{ mg}$$

Intramuscular administration is safer than IV administration which can result in anaphylaxis. The risk is highest with administration of Iron dextran complex (Imferon) and negligible for Iron sucrose complex. Intramuscular injections are given after hypersensitivity test for which 1 cc of drug is given I/M 24 hours before the regular injections.

Intravenous route is preferred over i/m where patient is noncompliant or there is no time for the total iron to be given by I/M route or patient has thrombocytopenia or injection abscess.

Oral iron is stopped before giving IV iron. Test dose is given with 1 ml of iron injection in 5 ml of syringe which is diluted to 5 ml with patient's venous blood after the venepucture. This has to be infused over a time of 5 minutes and patient should be carefully watched for allergy signs (headache, chest pain, hypotension, sweating, urticaria and rhonchi). Resuscitation tray should be ready and kept near the patient at time of infusion. One should wait for 24 hours before TDI to look for late reactions. Immediate reaction is anaphylaxis leading to respiratory and cardiac arrest, haemolysis and renal failure. Delayed reactions include myalgia, joint pains, skin rashes, lyphadenopathy, and thrombophlebitis at site of injection.

Q8. What is usual response to therapy?

The rate of increase in Hb is 0.1 g% per day irrespective of the route of administration. Significant rise in Hb is evident only after 2 to 3 weeks. The earliest response to therapy can be assessed by rise in reticulocyte count which becomes evident by 5–10 days.

Q9. If the anemia is not complicated by cardiac failure, do we still need to treat anemia?

Yes, anemia is a major cause of maternal and fetal mortality in India. Maternal complications associated with anemia are placental abruption, pre-eclampsia, preterm labour, UTI, puerperal sepsis and thromboembolism. Cardiac failure can result during third trimester, immediately after delivery and early puerperium. Fetal problems associated with anemia are spontaneous abortions, prematurity, fetal growth restrictions and fetal death. Infants born to severely anemic mothers are more likely to develop anemia and are more susceptible to infections.

Q10. What will you do if the patient is still anemic when she goes into labour?

Preferably a woman should have Hb level of at least 8 gm% before she goes in labour. The patient in labour should be propped up and given oxygen by mask, diuretics and antibiotic prophylaxis and digitalization if required. Packed cell transfusion should be given under diuretic cover. Intravenous fluids should be avoided to prevent fluid overload.

Intensive monitoring of vitals, periodic auscultation of chest for basal crepitations should be done throughout labour. Progress of labour is charted and minimal P/V examinations are done to avoid sepsis. Vaginal delivery is preferred unless there is obstetrical indication for caesarean section.

Second stage of labour should be cut short by forceps or ventouse application. Injection methergin for active management of third stage should be avoided. Instead inj oxytocin should be given for preventin of PPH. Active management of third stage should be done in all cases of anemia. Injection frusemide 40 mg, a diuretic, is given after delivery of placenta.

The patients of anemia are very sensitive to blood loss. The normal blood loss in vaginal delivery amounts to PPH in patient of severe anemia. One has to be vigilant and should treat PPH energetically with concentrated syntocinon and timely packed cell transfusions.

In cases complicated with anemia, iron therapy should continue atleast for 3 months after delivery and pregnancy should be avoided for a minimum of next 2 years.

Q11. If a woman comes with mild to moderate anemia in early gestation in OPD, how will you manage?

Depending on type of anemia, replacement therapy is given. National anemia control program recommends that for therapeutic use a dose of 100 mg elemental iron with 500 mcg folic acid should be given twice a day till Hb is normal and continued for another 12 weeks postpartum to replenish the iron stores.

Q12. How can you be sure if the patient is indeed taking oral iron therapy prescribed to her?

We find out if the patient is taking iron or not by asking the colour of her stool. With oral iron therapy, the stool turns black in colour.

CASE 3C PRE-ECLAMPSIA WITH BOH

A 30-year-old female $G_2P_1L_0$ presented to Antenatal clinic with h/o
Amenorrhea 32 weeks
Swelling over feet, face and hands × 1 week
No h/o fatigability, palpitations, orthopnea, PND
No h/o pain abdomen, leaking or bleeding per vaginum
Perceiving fetal movements adequately

HOPP: Booked and well supervised pregnancy
Ist antenatal visit in first trimester
Last antenatal visit 2 weeks back
No complications till then
Investigated, immunized and received iron prophylaxis

Obst history:
Ist pregnancy: Spontaneous conception, unsupervised unbooked pregnancy, h/o eclampsia at 8th month of gestation with IUD delivered vaginally 2 years back.
Was prescribed antihypertensives on discharge, discontinued at 2 weeks postpartum. Was normotensive thereafter.

Examination:
GC fair, afebrile, no pallor
Pulse: 80/min
BP: 150/100 mmHg
Pedal edema present
Chest/CVS: NAD
P/A: Abdominal wall edema present
Uterus: Fundal height 32 weeks
Single fetus, cephalic presentation, liquor adequate,
FHS: + 140/min, regular

Q1. What is pre-eclampsia?

Pre-eclampsia is a pregnancy-specific syndrome. It is a multisystem disorder associated with new-onset hypertension after 20 weeks of gestation associated with proteinuria.

The hypertension that develops as a consequence of pregnancy and regresses postpartum is called pregnancy-induced hypertension. It usually occurs after 20 weeks of gestation. However, it may also occur before 20 weeks in cases of hydatidiform mole. When the pregnancy-induced hypertension (see below) is associated with significant proteinuria (see below) and/or edema, it is called pre-eclampsia, and is associated with reduced organ perfusion secondary to vasospasm and endothelial activation. Pre-eclampsia superimposed with convulsions is referred as eclampsia.

Any of the following criteria is considered for diagnosing pregnancy-induced hypertension:

1. BP equal or more than 140/90 mmHg on two separate occasions at least 4 hour apart, or
2. MAP(mean arterial pressure) equal to or more than 105 mmHg, or
3. Systolic rise of 30 mmHg or more and a diastolic rise of 15 mmHg or more.

Significant proteinuria refers to

1. Urinary protein 1 g/L, 1+ or more on dipstick in two random urine samples collected 6 hr apart, or
2. 0.3 g/day in a 24 hour sample.

Q2. Why do you say that the above case is of mild pre-eclampsia? What are the criteria of severe pre-eclampsia?

Any one or more of the following features make it severe pre-eclampsia:

1. BP >160/110 mmHg;
2. Persistent 2+ or more proteinuria;

P/V Not done

Urine alb: 1+

Diagnosis: 30 years old, booked $G_2P_1L_0$ with 32 weeks pregnancy with mild pre-eclampsia with BOH

Investigations:

Blood group

Hb with platelet count

LFT with serum proteins

KFT with serum uric acid

GCT

24 hours urine protein

Fundus examination

USG for fetal biometry, amount of liquor and biophysical score

Non stress test

Adv:

Hospital admission

Bed rest

DFMR

w/f s/s of impending eclampsia, e.g. headache, blurring of vision, vomiting, rt hypochondriac pain

BP montoring 6 hourly

Urine albumin OD

Investigations (blood biochemistry weekly)

NST weekly

BPS fortnightly

Fetal biometry fortnightly

3. Signs and symptoms of impending eclampsia-nausea, vomiting, epigastric pain, headache, visual disturbance;
4. Pulmonary edema;
5. Oliguria;
6. HELLP syndrome (haemolysis, elevated liver enzymes, low platelet count);
7. FGR (fetal growth restriction) or oligohydramnios.

This patient has high BP with significant proteinuria (1+). Clinically there are no signs and symptoms of severe pre-eclampsia. Therefore clinical diagnosis is mild pre-eclampsia. However, only after the battery of investigations one can say that it is mild or severe pre-eclampsia.

Q3. In the obstetric history, you have used the word "spontaneous conception". Do you mean "unplanned conception"?

No, spontaneous conception means conception without any infertility treatment.

Q4. In P/A examination, you mention "abdominal wall edema absent". Do you actually mean "abdominal wall edema" or do you mean "ascites"?

I mean abdominal wall edema. Pedal edema of pregnancy is very common and is considered physiological. However, if it occurs on abnormal sites, e.g abdomen, hands and face and persists even after rest, it is considered pathological. In pre-eclampsia there is edema in the non-dependant parts like face, hands, abdominal wall, etc.

Q5. In history, you have asked about pain abdomen, leaking or bleeding P/V. Did you ask these questions as a routine or are these questions particularly important to this case?

As the patient has presented in third trimester history of pain abdomen and leaking is taken to know whether patient is in labour or not. History of bleeding P/V is asked as a routine to rule out antepartum hemorrhage especially in pre-eclampsia where abruption is more common.

Q6. The case sheet says: P/V not done. Is there a special reason why it is not done?

As the patient is not in labour and there is no indication for immediate termination of pregnancy, a P/V examination is not indicated.

Q7. You have advised weekly NST. What is meant by NST?

NST stands for non-stress test. It is the most commonly used test for assessment for fetal well-being in antenatal period. This test is based on the premise that the heart rate of a fetus who is not acidotic as a result of hypoxia will temporarily accelerate in response to fetal movements. Normal NST is two or more accelerations that peak at 15 beats per min or more above baseline, each lasting 15 seconds or more (Fig. 3.1). The duration of test is 20 minutes. This test involves use of Doppler to detect fetal heart rate and maternal perception of the fetal movements. Normal NST is reported as reactive NST and if these criteria are not met it is reported as nonreactive.

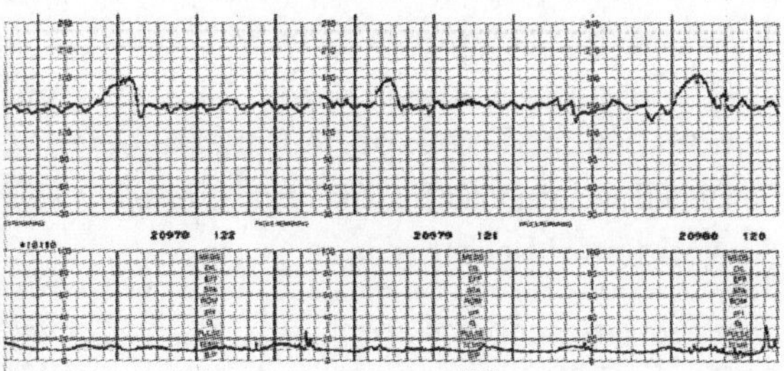

Fig. 3.1: Normal (reactive) NST

Q8. Is the management of this case any different from that of normal pregnancy?

Delivery is the only cure for this disease and the goal of management is to ensure that pregnancy continues uneventfully till the 37th week when the pregnancy is terminated and a healthy baby is delivered. Most of the patients with pre-eclampsia need admission in the hospital. Such a management plan requires control of hypertension, early diagnosis and prompt treatment of the complications. It includes rest, regular diet without strict salt restriction, maternal and fetal monitoring, and antihypertensives. No diuretics and sedatives are given unless there is pulmonary edema. If everything goes uneventful, pregnancy is terminated at 37 completed weeks.

Q9. How will you manage the hypertension in this patient?

The aim of treating high BP during pregnancy is to avoid complications due to hypertension *per se*, it does not alter the course of the disease. Drug treatment is recommended if the maternal blood pressure exceeds 160/100 mmHg.

The drug of choice in pregnancy is methyl dopa 250 mg bd and can be increased to a maximum dose of 1 g tds. The usual dose given is 500 mg qid. If the BP is still not controlled it is prudent to add a second drug with different mechanism of action, e.g. nifedipine (calcium channel blocker) 10 mg bd. Methyl dopa is used as the first line drug because of it's safety profile in pregnancy. An antihypertensive medication to be avoided during pregnancy is angiotensin-converting enzyme (ACE) inhibitors, as they are associated with fetal renal dysgenesis or death when used in the second and third trimesters. Angiotensin II receptor antagonists/blockers are not used during pregnancy because of similar effects as ACE inhibitors. Diuretics do not cause fetal malformations but are generally avoided in pregnancy as they prevent the physiologic volume expansion seen in normal pregnancy. They may be used in states of volume-dependant hypertension, such as renal or cardiac disease.

Q10. Can there be any complication while the patient is under medical supervision?

There is increased maternal morbidity and mortality due to convulsions (eclampsia), cerebral haemorrhage, pulmonary edema, visual disturbances, renal and hepatic dysfunction, and HELLP syndrome. Eclampsia is mostly preceded by severe pre-eclampsia, however it can be superim-posed on mild pre-eclampsia. Increased perinatal morbidity and mortality is due to FGR, accidental haemorrhage and prematurity.

Q11. What is HELLP syndrome?

HELLP syndrome is a life-threatening obstetric complication usually considered to be a variant of pre-eclampsia. Both conditions occur during the later stages of pregnancy, or sometimes after childbirth. HELLP is an abbreviation of the main findings, viz.

1. Hemolytic anemia,
2. Elevated liver enzymes and
3. Low platelet count.

Q12. Can patients of PIH be managed on outdoor basis?

Ambulatory treatment can be offered to patients of nonproteinuric hypertension or mild pre-eclampsia with 1+ urine albumin, provided patient is compliant and can contact the doctor or hospital if need arises in emergency hours.

Patient is advised to daily record BP, urine albumin, maternal weight DFMR. Patient should be informed about s/s of severe pre-eclampsia. She should report to the hospital if –BP >140/90 mmHg, Vaginal bleeding, urine alb>1+, S/S of Severe PE. During ambulatory management patient has to report weekly for biochemical surveillance

Patient is hospitalized if there is any evidence of disease progression for mother (acute exacerbation of HT or proteinuria, s/s or lab finding of severe PE) or Fetal compromise (oligohydramnios, fetal growth restriction, abnormal wave forms).

Q13. How will you manage if this patient develops severe pre-eclampsia?

At 32 weeks we would like to wait for fetal maturity of at least 34 weeks provided patients condition is stable. The patient is therefore shifted to the labour room for intensive monitoring which includes Maternal evaluation (General condition, coagulation profile, LFT, KFT, Output monitoring), prophylactic anticonvulsant ($MgSO_4$), antihypertensives, Proper fluid therapy and foetal evaluation (NST, BPS, Doppler). Steroid (Betamethasone) is also given to enhance lung maturity in fetus.

Q14. What will you do if the pre-eclampsia cannot be controlled?

In such cases, we terminate the pregnancy. There are both maternal and fetal indications for terminating the pregnancy. The maternal indications of termination of pregnancy are:

1. Eclampsia
2. S/s of impending eclampsia
3. Severe pre-eclampsia after 34 weeks
4. Severe pre-eclampsia before 34 weeks and not stabilized on expectant management
5. Papilloedema on fundus examination, and
6. Accidental haemorrhage.

The fetal indications are:

1. Severe FGR or severe oligohydramnios;
2. Abnormal NST with abnormal BPS.

Q15. As this patient had previous history of eclampsia, is she more prone to have pre-eclamsia in this pregnancy? Can we prevent it?

Women who develop pre-eclampsia/eclampsia during pregnancy have an increased risk of recurrent pre-eclampsia during subsequent pregnancies. The overall risk is about 10–18%. The risk is higher in women who develop severe early pre-eclampsia (i.e. before 27 weeks' gestation).

Multiple interventions to prevent pre-eclampsia have been investigated. These include low-dose acetylsalicylic acid (ASA), supplemental calcium, salt restriction, supplemental magnesium, and fish oil therapy. While several large trials of ASA in high-risk populations showed minimal benefit in reducing the frequency of pre-eclampsia, a recent meta-analysis reported an approximate 15% reduction in pre-eclampsia among pregnant women taking low-dose ASA. This therapy appears very safe and might be considered in high-risk women. None of the other therapies have demonstrated any significant preventive benefit. One recent trial demonstrated some preventive benefit to supplemental antioxidants (vitamins C and E), but these results remain to be confirmed. This patient might have benefited with 75 mg ASA given from early pregnancy till 34 weeks.

CASE 3D INTRAUTERINE GROWTH RESTRICTION

$G_1P_0A_0$ reported to the antenatal clinic with complaints of 32 weeks amenorrhoea

HOPP: Registered pregnancy with infrequent antenatal visits. First visit at 8 weeks, pregnancy confirmed by UPT followed by USG examination.

Last visit 2 months back

Received TT immunization and iron prophylaxis

No h/o any complications in any trimesters

Obst history: Primigravida

Menstrual history: MC: 5/28–32 days, regular, normal

No significant past medical, surgical, family history

Dietary history: Diet adequate in calories and proteins

Examination:

GC Fair
Weight: 54 kg, Height: 5ft 2inches
Pallor: nil
Pulse: 80/min, regular
BP: 120/80 mmHg
No pedal oedema
Chest/ CVS: NAD

P/A

Uterus enlarged, fundal height: 28 weeks (measurements: fundal height: 25 cm; abdominal girth at umbilicus: 24 inches)
Single fetus, longitudinal lie with cephalic presentation,
Liquor clinically less
FHS: 140/min regular

Diagnosis

A 30-year-old $G_1P_0A_0$ with 32 weeks pregnancy with suspected growth restriction

Q1. What is intrauterine growth restriction (IUGR)?

Low birth weight infants who are small for gestational age are designated to be suffering from fetal growth restriction. Intrauterine fetal growth restriction is defined as fetal weight or abdominal circumference below the tenth percentile for that gestational age. The term fetal growth retardation has been discarded now because "retardation" implies mental subnormality.

IUGR is generally differentiated into symmetrical or asymmetrical. Fetal growth restriction may be symmetrical when there is proportionate reduction in the size of all body parts (BPD, FL and AC, all are less than normal). It is usually very early onset and mostly caused by fetal factors like structural or chromosomal anomalies or congenital infections. Asymmetrical IUGR often occurs late in third trimester–late onset IUGR due to maternal diseases causing placental insufficiency. In this type fetal head size is normal while abdominal circumference is reduced.

Q2. Does it make sense to calculate the gestational age from the fetal length? How can we be sure that there is no IUGR?

IUGR does not start in the first trimester. The crown rump length in first trimester is the most accurate way of determining gestational age with error of only 2–3 days. USG is usually done in first trimester for determining exact gestational age in women who are not sure of LMP dates or in high-risk pregnancy like diabetes where elective termination may be required at term and thus knowledge of gestational age will be important to avoid preterm termination.

In case of non-availability of first trimester USG, P/V findings in 1st trimester can be used for calculating period of gestation. P/V in the first trimester/CRL in 1st trimester (whatever available) is the most accurate method for dating. Next, we observe the weight gain in pregnancy. In 1st trimester she does not gain any weight. The fetus does not increase in size very much and she may lose weight due to vomiting. It is mainly in the 2nd and 3rd trimester that she gains weight. It is 4lbs or 1 Kg per month on an average. When weight gain during antenatal visits is adequate and her fundal height corresponds to the gestational age calculated from LMP (Ist trimester USG or P/V examination if dates unsure or mistaken), we are reasonably sure that IUGR is not there.

Abdominal palpation is an important tool for screening of IUGR. IUGR is suspected when on clinical examination fundal height is less than period of gestation and the difference is >4 weeks. Preferably symphyseal fundal height measurement should be done on antenatal examination. The SFH measurement corresponds to weeks of gestation +2 cm after 24 weeks to 36 weeks, and 3 cm from 36–42 weeks. A discrepancy of 3 cm or more is suggestive of IUGR.

Q3. What would you do if fundal height does not correspond to gestational age?

We shall first confirm IUGR by doing an ultrasound. May be, the patient gave a wrong date of LMP. Sometimes in symmetrical IUGR it may not be possible to diagnose growth restriction by single USG especially if gestational age is not sure. In such cases repeat USG is required to see the growth velocity and thus diagnosis of IUGR.

Once IUGR is diagnosed we have to look for causes like inadequate maternal diet, maternal disease, fetal congenital defects, chromosomal anomalies, or fetal infections. If none exists, we have to do fetal surveillance and depending on fetal growth and fetal assessment test results decide the appropriate time for termination of pregnancy.

Adv

Investigations:

USG: Fetal biometry to diagnose IUGR, congenital anomalies, amount of liquor, placental localization and grading.

USG findings: Asymmetrical IUGR, Liquor reduced (AFI-5 cm), placenta upper segment grade 2, No GCA

Once diagnosed on USG, other tests done simultaneously on USG

Biophysical scoring and NST

Doppler flow studies: Umbilical artery S/D ratio

Routine tests: Hb, blood group, VDRL, GCT, TSH, HIV testing after counseling

Tests to find cause of IUGR:

Anomaly scan on USG

Lupus anticoagulant and anticardiolipin antibodies

TORCH

Urine: R/M and culture

Results: BPS: 8/8, NST: reactive

Umbilical artery blood flow: Normal

All other tests normal

Management:

Admit

Bed rest

DFMR

Inj betamethasone 12 mg I/M 2 doses 24 hours apart

Fetal monitoring: NST: twice in a week, BPS and Doppler weekly

Fetal growth 2 weekly by clinical examination and USG biometry

If monitoring remains normal, patient can be discharged and monitored as outdoor patient.

Q4. How does an ultrasound help you to confirm IUGR?

Previous USG is used for gestational age dating especially if first trimester USG is available. When clinical suspicion of IUGR is there USG is done to confirm IUGR by fetal measurements. Fetal measurements taken on USG are BPD (biparital diameter) or HC (head circumference), FL (femur length) and AC (abdominal circumference). We check whether these measurements are corresponding to the gestational age or lagging behind. If BPD and FL corresponds with gestational age and abdominal circumference is small for gestational age, this indicates asymmetrical IUGR. However, if all the three parameters are corresponding with each other but are smaller than the gestational age, then 3 possibilities exist:

i. It can be wrong dates,
ii. It can be a constitutionally small baby, or
iii. It can be symmetrical IUGR. The first can be confirmed by accurate dating of pregnancy. To differentiate (ii) and (iii), we have to do serial ultrasound (every week) to know the growth potential. If growth velocity is normal, it favors the constitutionally small baby or else, it is SFD (small-for-dates) fetus.

Once IUGR is diagnosed on fetal biometry on USG, a set of investigations are done to find the cause after detailed history and examination to look for maternal diseases.

Q5. How do you manage IUGR if all investigations are normal?

Little can be done to treat fetal growth restriction and therefore in most cases, the only option open to the obstetrician is to deliver the baby. The biggest challenge is to deliver at the optimum time so as to minimize the damage to the baby both from intrauterine factors and from prematurity. Fetal well-being is judged by fetal surveillance tests. In mild IUGR, if the tests results are normal, the patient can be managed as outdoor patient with weekly surveillance. The frequency of testing is generally weekly/twice weekly NST and BPS and weekly Doppler studies and fortnightly biometry. If test results are abnormal, delivery is planned considering fetal maturity versus test abnormality. If delivery is required before 34 weeks, injection Betamethasone is given to enhance fetal lung maturity before delivery.

Q6. What is the optimum time to deliver such a baby?

Delivery is planned considering fetal surveillance test results and fetal maturity. Factors to be considered are: what are the risks to fetus if pregnancy is continued vs survival risks after delivery because of prematurity. If the fetus is 28 weeks old, its chances of survival in the nursery is only 50%. Therefore we try to prolong the pregnancy with intensive fetal surveillance at least up to 34 weeks if fetal well-being tests permit. The patient must be informed of all this before taking any step. Delivery is indicated irrespective of maturity when a single or a combination of the surveillance tests indicate imminent fetal danger and the fetal risk from a hostile intrauterine environment is judged to be greater than that from pulmonary maturity. Delivery is recommended in IUGR fetus in following situations:

a. When all surveillance findings including umbilical flow are normal, delay delivery until at least 37 weeks.
b. When end diastolic flow is absent or reversed or amniotic fluid is decreased.
c. If there is abnormal NST (decelerations with reduced variability) or abnormal BPS (≤4), deliver at 34 weeks even if other tests are normal.

If termination of pregnancy is required at 34 weeks (preterm), the mode of delivery has to be according to the fetal condition on surveillance tests and cervical scoring. Cesarean delivery is indicated in a preterm fetus in

a. Severely compromised fetus (BPS ≤4),
b. Severe Oligohydramnios, and
c. Poor Bishop score of cervix.

If cervix is favorable, labour induction with oxytocin is to be done. During labour, monitoring has to be done as for any high risk labour. Intrapartum monitoring with continuous CTG is recommended.

Delivery should be done in a unit where optimal neonatal expertise and care facilities are available. Before going ahead with delivery at ≤34 weeks, antenatal steroids (Inj beta-methasone 12 mg I/M 12 hourly) should be given to the mother and induction of labour/LSCS should be planned 24 hours later to prevent respiratory distress syndrome in the premature neonate.

Q7. What are the investigations done once IUGR is diagnosed?

Once IUGR is diagnosed we do

- Level II USG in which we look for
  i. Major congenital anomalies,
  ii. Features suggestive of fetal infections like intracranial calcification, microcephaly, hepatosplenomegaly, etc. and
  iii. Any Placental causes.
- Umbilical artery Doppler study is done to assess fetoplacental circulation.
- Toxoplasma, Rubella, Cytomegalovirus antibody testing (TORCH) is done in maternal blood to detect fetoplacental infections.
- Testing for urinary tract infection (Urine c/s) should be done.
- To detect antiphospholipid syndrome, Lupus anticoagulant and anticardiolipin antibodies testing should be done.

CASE 3E ANTEPARTUM HEMORRHAGE

A 28-year-old $G_2P_1L_1$
c/o Amenorrhoea 34 weeks
c/o Bleeding p/v around 500 cc few hours back
Bleeding was painless, started suddenly when she was asleep (causeless)
Bleeding stopped after one episode
No h/o any trauma
No h/o labour pains or leaking P/v
Perceiving fetal movements adequately

HOPP: Unbooked unsupervised pregnancy
Pregnancy diagnosed by fetal movements at 4 months
Only two visits in dispensary for TT immunization
No investigations done

Obst history: $G_2P_1L_1$
Ist: LSCS at term for breech presentation 2 years back, baby A&H
No complications in antepartum or postpartum
Lactated for 1.5 years

Menstrual history: Had periods only twice since after last child birth, conceived in lactational period
No contraception used

O/E:
Pallor: Moderate
Pulse: 92/min, reg
BP: 110/70 mmHg
Pedal oedema +
Chest/CVS: NAD
P/A: Uterus enlarged, fundal height 32 weeks, single fetus, transverse lie
FHS: 130/min, regular

Q1. What is antepartum hemorrhage and what are its causes?

Antepartum hemorrhage is defined as genital tract bleeding after 20 weeks of pregnancy till anytime before the third stage of labour. It usually occurs in the third trimester.

The causes of APH can be placental or extraplacental. The majority of cases have placental causes, with placenta previa being the commonest. Extraplacental causes, e.g. cervical pathology or growth in vagina, are not common.

The normal site of placental implantation is in the upper segment of the uterus. If it encroaches on to the lower segment, it is called placenta previa. Diagnosis is made antenatally by USG examination. On USG internal os is visualized and measure the distance between lower edge of placenta and internal os. If it is <5 cm then it is encroaching on the lower uterine segment. Lower uterine segment is approximately up to 5 cm above internal os.

The second major cause is *abruptio placentae*, which we also call as *accidental hemorrhage* due to premature separation of normally situated placenta which can be concealed, (i.e. when there is a retroplacental clot, uterus becomes tense and tender, immediately and invariably there is fetal distress/death) as well as revealed (i.e. when blood flows out). If we do not detect concealed hemorrhage in time, the patient can develop DIC, renal failure and hemorrhagic shock.

Q2. If the placenta is normally placed early in pregnancy, can there be a placenta previa later?

If the placenta is in the upper segment earlier, there is little chance that it will shift to the lower segment. However, the reverse is not true: If the placenta is in the lower segment, there can be *placental migration* (The term is a misnomer as the placenta does not migrate. Rather, the uterus gets enlarged so that the lower margin of the placenta is away from the os.) If the placenta covers the os (*central placenta previa*), there is less chance that it will migrate. If the placenta is in the lower segment of the uterus with the lower border away from the os in early pregnancy, the chances are that it will be in the upper segment in 3rd trimester. If it is in upper segment in mid-trimester, it usually remains there.

Q3. How early in pregnancy can the location of the placenta be ascertained, and by what method?

Location of placenta can be ascertained in second trimester of pregnancy by USG examination.

Q4. You have advised USG with Doppler to look for Placenta accreta/percreta. What are placenta acreta/percreta?

Placenta accreta is an abnormally firm attachment of the placenta to the uterine wall. When the placenta invades the partial thickness of myometrium it is called placenta increta and when it invades the entire thickness of the myometrium to breach the serosa, it is called placenta percreta. Placenta accreta is quite common in placenta previa, especially when placenta previa is implanted anteriorly in a patient delivered by Cesarean section in a previous pregnancy. The risk is less in this case since the placenta is posterior. However, a color Doppler ultrasound is performed in all women with placenta previa to rule out placenta accreta.

Q5. How would you approach a case of APH if you do not have ultrasound facilities?

To confirm the diagnosis in the absence of USG facilities, a digital vaginal examination is done in the OT with full preparedness for general anesthesia and Caesarean section, since it carries the risk of torrential bleeding.

Uterus relaxed, neither tense nor tender
L/E: No bleeding p/v

Adv: USG for placental localization and retroplacental hemorrhage along with routine parameters like gestational age, amount of liquor and congenital anomalies.

USG: Single live fetus 32 weeks in transverse lie, no GCA, liquor adequate, placenta posterior covering the os, No RPC

Diagnosis: $G_2P_1L_1$ with 32 weeks pregnancy with placenta previa (type 3) with APH with anemia with previous cesarean section.

Investigations and management:
HmG with P/S for type of anemia
Blood group
GCT
HIV testing
Urine r/m
USG with Doppler to look for placenta accreta/percreta

Admit in the hospital and keep under observation
Bed rest
Treat anemia
Arrange 1 unit blood
Inj Betamethasone 12 mg i/m 2 doses 24 hours apart
w/f vitals, fetal monitoring, bleeding per vaginum

If no further bleeding episode: Elective LSCS after 37 weeks
If recurrent bleeding episodes with stable condition: LSCS after 34 weeks.
If excessive bleeding, fetal distress: Emergency LSCS irrespective of gestational age.

This is known as the Double set up examination. This is done in cases with gestation >38 weeks or when patient is bleeding and mode of termination has to be decided.

During the P/V, all four vaginal fornices are felt: (i) If there is soft tissue between the examining finger and the fetal skull, then placenta previa is diagnosed. (ii) If the fetal skull is easily felt in all four fornices, then a careful examination is done through the cervix. (iii) If placental tissue is felt, then a caesarean section should be done. If not, the membranes can be ruptured with the aim of allowing a vaginal delivery.

Q6. What would you do if a routine USG examination early in pregnancy shows a placenta previa?

In most cases, the position of the placenta changes in relation to the internal os of the cervix as pregnancy continues and therefore, a follow-up ultrasound examination must be arranged after the gestational age of 32–34 weeks.

Q7. Can APH be prevented if the placenta previa is detected early?

Not really, since most of the time, the bleeding in placenta previa occurs without any external cause. When the placenta is located over internal os, the formation of the lower uterine segment and dilatation of the internal os inevitably result in the tearing of placental attachments. The bleeding is augmented by the inability of the myometrial fibres of the lower uterine segment to contract and thereby constrict the torn vessels. Nonetheless, the patient is advised restricted activity and kept on expectant management with planning of termination at 37 weeks.

Q8. What are important steps in the management of antepartum haemorrhage?

The management consists of 4 important steps that should be carried out in the following order:

1. The maternal condition must be evaluated and stabilized, if necessary.
2. The condition of the fetus must then be assessed.
3. The cause of the haemorrhage must be diagnosed.
4. Finally, the definitive management of an antepartum haemorrhage, depending on the cause, must be given.

It must also be decided whether the patient should be transferred for further treatment.

Q9. Do you always do cesarean in cases of placent aprevia?

Class I and II anterior may be able to deliver vaginally; Grades II posterior, III and IV will require caesarean section by a senior obstetrician. This patient will require caesarean section.

Q10. Does the bleeding stop after delivery?

No. Patients with placenta previa also have an increased risk of *postpartum* haemorrhage because the lower uterine segment does not have the same ability as the upper segment to contract and retract after delivery. It is therefore important to watch for PPH in these cases.

CASE 3F PRETERM LABOUR

$G_2P_{0+1+0+0}$ with 32 weeks pregnancy
C/o intermittent pain abdomen every half hr for 3–4 hours
No h/o leaking/bleeding/discharge P/V
No urinary complaints
Booked supervised pregnancy
Antenatal period uneventful

Past obstetrical history:
Ist: Preterm vaginal delivery at 30 weeks, labour pains followed by delivery at home, unsupervised, uneventful pregnancy. Baby died after few hours. 2 years back

Past medical history, family history, uneventful

Dietary history: Adequate

O/E: GC Fair
Pulse: 80 mmHg, BP: 120/80 mmHg
Pallor: mild
No pedal oedema

Chest/ CVS: NAD

P/A: Uterus 30–32 weeks,
Single fetus, Longitudinal lie
Cephalic presentation
FHS: 140/min, regular
Mild Uterine Contractions present
20 sec/30–40 min

P/V: Cervix 2 cm dilated, 50% effaced
Vertex at –3, membranes present,
BOM forming
Pelvis adequate

Diagnosis: Booked $G_2P_{0+1+0+0}$ with 32 weeks pregnancy with preterm labour without PROM

Q1. Why did you diagnose this case as preterm labour?

Preterm labour is diagnosed between 20–37 weeks if labour pains are present with following criteria:

1. Uterine contractions 4 in 20 min or 8 in 60 min associated with progressive cervical change;
2. Dilatation of cervix >1 cm; and
3. Effacement 80% or more. In the present case antenatal woman is having uterine contractions with cervical dilatation of 2 cm, and therefore she is diagnosed as having preterm labour.

Q2. Among the investigations, why did you include an ultrasound?

Obstetric ultrasound is done to rule out any cause like fetal, placental, liquor abnormalities where delivery may be preferable.

On USG we look for fetal maturity, growth abnormalities, anomalies, placental localization and maturity, amount of liquor, etc.

Q3. Should tocolysis be given to all patients with preterm labour?

Tocolytics are given in case of preterm labour without PPROM with gestation <34 weeks. There is no need to prevent or delay labour in gestations >34 weeks, as morbidity/mortality is very low after 34 weeks. Tocolysis has no effect if patient is in active labour, i.e. cervical dilatation ≥3 cm. In certain situations tocolytics are contraindicated as we will like delivery to occur. These include severe eclampsia/pre-eclampsia, placental abruption, advanced cervical dilatation, and evidence of fetal compromise.

Q4. What is BPP?

The BPP (biophysical profile) combines 5 parameters:

1. The nonstress test (NST),

Adv:
Admit in labour room
Bed rest
I/V fluids: 500 ml of RL
Inj. Betamethasone 12 mg I/M 12 hourly for 2 doses
Nifedipine 20 mg oral, repeat after 30 min if required followed by 10–20 mg 6 hourly
W/f pulse, BP, uterine contractions, leaking P/V

Investigations:
HmG
Urine C/S
HVS C/S
USG for fetal maturity, fetal growth parameters, anomalies, liquor amount, placental localization
Shift to ward once contractions have subsided.
Fetal surveillance tests: BPS and NST
Discontinue nifedipine after 48 hours if contractions have subsided.

2. Ultrasound measurement of the AFV,
3. Observation of the presence or absence of fetal breathing movements,
4. Gross body movements, and
5. *Tone*

   These data are obtained from 2 sources, i.e. ultrasound imaging and fetal heart rate monitoring.

Q5. Why did you prescribe steroids?

Antenatal corticosteroids are indicated in all women between 24 and 34 weeks of gestation with preterm labour. Steroid induces lung maturity and prevents RDS in preterm newborn, decreases intraventricular hemorrhage, and decreases necrotizing enterocolitis.

Q6. Why did you prescribe nifedipine?

Nifedipine is a tocolytic. It is given to inhibit uterine contractions in gestations <34 weeks. Tocolytics are generally given for 48 hours. Long term tocolysis is not useful.

Q7. Can you predict preterm labour? Are there warning signs? Can we prevent preterm labour?

In majority of the cases, preterm labour can't be predicted though its chances are higher if there is a prior history of preterm delivery. However, there are some warning signs for preterm labour in antenatal patients. These include menstruation-like cramps, low dull backache, mucoid vaginal discharge, feeling of pelvic pressure or heaviness in vagina, and bacterial vaginosis. Asymtomatic cervical dilatation or shortening of cervix <2.5 cm (detected on USG) or presence of fetal fibronectin in cervicovaginal secretions are useful in symptomatic cases to predict which of them will deliver preterm. However, these tests are not useful for predicting preterm labour in asymptomatic women. Progesterone, though a weak tocolytic, has been found to be useful in preventing preterm labour. It is given as 250 mg 17α hydroxypregesterone I/M weekly or 100 mg natural progesterone vaginally daily.

Q8. What would you do if a woman with uterine contractions does not show cervical change?

Such cases need to be observed. If there is no cervical change, there is no immediate need for treatment. To predict whether she is likely to develop preterm labour later, we would do

1. An USG for cervical length and internal os dilatation; and
2. Fetal fibronectin in cervicovaginal secretion. If cervical length is <2.5 cm, internal os is dilated >1 cm or fetal

fibronectin is detected in cervical secretions, there are high chances that the woman would deliver prematurely. In such case, we would give steroids to the patient and shift her to the hospital. Progesterone should be given for preventing preterm labour till 34 weeks.

Q9. Does the plan of management change if leaking P/V is also present?

Yes, if preterm labour is associated with leaking of amniotic fluid then labour is not inhibited with tocolytics. Injectable antibiotic are started in these case. When membranes are ruptured, there is risk of ascending infection from lower genital tract and labour is generally a marker of subclinical infection. Therefore labour is not inhibited in such cases except in a few situations when patient has to be transferred to a higher centre for delivery. In such cases, utmost care has to be taken to rule out intrauterine infection before giving tocolytics for a very short term only for transfer (Ref Case 3G).

Q10. How is preterm delivery managed?

In first stage of labour, bedrest is given so as to preserve the membranes as long as possible. Minimum P/V examination is done. When the membranes rupture, rule out cord prolapse because the preterm head fits poorly in the lower segment, increasing the chances of cord prolapse. Sedation is avoided and therefore epidural analgesia is given for pain relief. Antibiotic prophylaxis for neonatal sepsis with group B streptococcal infection is given during labour. During the second stage, liberal episiotomy is given. Instrumental delivery is avoided but if required, forceps are used. Ventouse is never applied on the preterm head. The cord is clamped immediately on delivery. The management of third stage is the same as in normal labour.

CASE 3G PRETERM PREMATURE RUPTURE OF MEMBRANES

$G_2P_0A_1$ with 30 weeks amenorrhoea
C/o watery discharge per vaginum × 3 hours
No h/o labour pains
No h/o bleeding P/V
Antenatal period uneventful
Booked supervised pregnancy, received two doses of TT

Past obst history
MTP at 12 weeks pregnancy 1 year back (Ind. Contraceptive failure). MTP done with suction evacuation.
No other significant history

O/E: GC fair
Afebrile
Pulse: 82/min
BP: 120/80 mmHg
No pedal oedema
Chest/CVS: NAD

P/A: Uterus 28 weeks, single fetus, cephalic presentation
Liquor decreased clinically
FHS+ regular, 140/min
No uterine tenderness

P/S: Clear watery discharge from cervical os seen on coughing
Cervix long, external os closed

Diagnosis: $G_2P_0A_1$, with 30 weeks gestation with PPROM.

Adv
Admit labour room for observation
Bedrest
W/f pulse, temperature, uterine contractions, uterine tenderness, FHS, amount of leaking and color/smell of liquor

Q1. What is PPROM?

Preterm prelabour rupture of membranes (PPROM) defined as rupture of membranes at least 1 hour prior to the onset of labour at less than 37 weeks gestation. It precedes 1/3rd of preterm labours.

Q2. How do you diagnose rupture of membranes?

Diagnosis is certain when a history of sudden gush of watery discharge is there and on examination, amniotic fluid is observed draining from cervix on perspeculum examination. If in doubt, one can differentiate amniotic fluid from cervicovaginal discharge by performing

1. The *nitrazine testing* of vaginal discharge pH (amniotic fuid is alkaline) and
2. *Ferning test* (microscopic inspection of secretions shows ferning pattern due to NaCl crystallization). Both tests have high false positive rate. USG detection of decreased liquor also helps in reaching the diagnosis of PPROM in doubtful cases.

P/V examination should not be done if the woman is not in labour.

Q3. Can PPROM lead to any complications?

Yes, a major complication is peterm delivery with the associated neonatal complications of prematurity. It can also lead to intrauterine infections (chrioamnionitis, endometritis, maternal wound infections and neonatal sepsis), cord compression and cord prolapse, and abruption.

Q4. How do you diagnose chorioamnionitis?

The patient may have fever, tachycardia, uterine tenderness and foul smelling vaginal discharge. Fetal tachycardia also is warning sign of chorioamnionitis. Labouratory evidence of increased TLC, c-reactive proteins and positive cultures substantia the diagnosis.

Q5. How would you manage a case of PPROM?

If a case of PPROM presents with premature onset of labour, the labour is allowed to proceed in a tertiary care centre with good neonatal care facilities. Even if PPROM is not associated with labour pains, the patient is admitted to the labour room for observation, especially for s/s of infection (fever, tachycardia, uterine tenderness, and yellowish foul-smelling discharge).

If there is no s/s of infection and no fetal compromise, such conservative management is continued till 34 weeks whereafter labour is induced. Labour is induced earlier if there is chorioamnionitis or fetal compromise. A cesarean section is indicated if

a. There is severe oligohydramnios with almost no liquor,
b. Cord prolapse, or
c. Severe fetal compromise with unfavorable cervix.

In absence of infection, we try to delay the delivery to 34 weeks as survival of the fetus improves with every passing week. After 34 weeks, morbidity and mortality is very rare, and therefore delivery is not delayed. In extreme prematurity <24 weeks, conservative management is done only in cases in which there is autosealing of the defect in the membranes and the leaking stops, else, labour is induced.

Investigations
HmG
C-Reactive protein
Urine c/s
HVS c/s
USG: Amount of liquor
BPS
Investigations: Normal
USG: Single live fetus, maturity by BPD, FL, AC is 30±1 weeks, placenta posterior upper segment, grade 2, liquor decreased, only single pocket of 1 cm seen
NST: Reactive
BPS: 10/10

Plan: Conservative management
Observe for chorioamnionitis clinically and by alternate day testing if leaking continues
Oral erythromycin 500 mg QID × 10 days
Inj betamethasone 12 mg I/M 12 hourly × 2 doses
If no S/S of infection, continue this till 34 weeks
BPS biweekly

4 Delivery of the Fetus and Labour Room Procedures

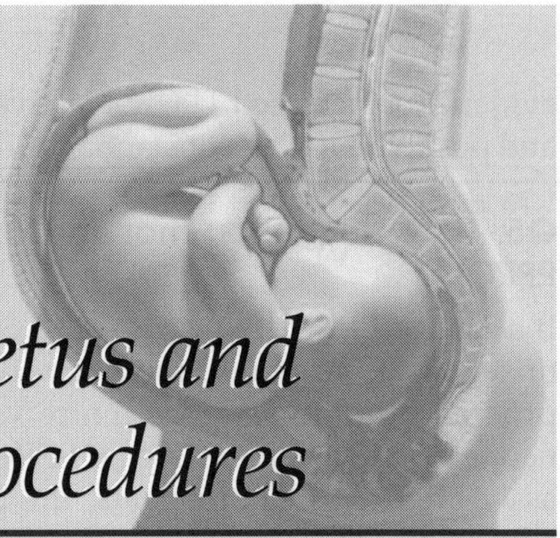

> **CASE 4A**
> **NORMAL VAGINAL DELIVERY**
>
> Mrs X, 24 years old, Primigravida
> c/o 38 weeks amenorrhoea
> labour pains × 4 hours
> passage of blood mixed disharge p/v
> No h/o leaking or bleeding p/v
> HOPP: Booked, supervised pregnancy, immunized, antenatal period uneventful
> LMP: 22.09.2007
> EDD: 29.06.2008
> POG: 38 weeks (on 15.06.08)
> No significant past medical or surgical history
> *O/E:* GC fair
> Pallor: Mild
> Pulse: 80/min, regular
> BP: 120/80 mmHg
> No pedal oedema
> Chest & CVS: NAD
> P/A: Uterus term size
> Mild contractions present 20 sec/5 min
> Singleton fetus, longitudinal lie
> Cephalic 3/5th above brim
> FHS +nt, 140/min, regular
> Liquor adequate

Q1. You have diagnosed that the woman is in the latent phase of labour. What is latent phase of labour?

There are 4 stages of labour:

Stage 1: From onset of true labour pains till full dilatation of cervix (10 cm). It is further sub-divided into:

a. The *latent phase,* which commences with the maternal perception of regular contractions and slow cervical dilatation and ends with a cervical dilatation of 3 cm. The latent phase should not be longer than 8 hours.
b. The *active phase,* which starts from a cervical diameter of 3 cm to the full cervical dilatation of 10 cm. For normal progress of labour, the rate of cervical dilatation should be >1 to 1.2 cm/hour in the nulliparous, and >1.5 cm/hour in multiparous women. The active phase should not last longer than 12 hours. Most labour abnormalities occur in this phase and therefore this phase is closely monitored for progress of labour.

Stage 2: From full dilatation of cervix till the delivery of the baby.

Stage 3: From delivery of the baby to expulsion of placenta and membranes.

Stage 4: After delivery of placenta. This is the stage of monitoring for 1 hour as life threatening complication of PPH is more likely at this time.

In the present case, the patient is in latent phase because cervical dilatation is <3 cm.

P/V: cervix 2.5 cm dilated, 75% effaced, membranes intact, BOM forming, Vx at –2 station, LOA position
Pelvis adequate
Diagnosis: 24 years booked primigravida with 38 weeks pregnancy with singleton live fetus with cephalic presentation in latent phase of labour

Q2. How can you be sure that an abdominal pain is a labour pain?

Labour pains are painful uterine contractions that can be easily identified by their characteristics: They are intermittent with pain-free intervals, start from the back and radiate to the front, and their intensity and frequency increase with time.

A clinical sign associated with labour pains is the intermittent hardening and relaxation of the uterus. The hardening of the uterus, felt per-abdominally, precedes and outlasts the pain. The pain occurs only when the intensity of uterine contraction exceeds a threshold.

Q3. What causes false labour pains? How do you differentiate them from true labour pains?

False labour pains, like true labour pains, are associated with uterine contractions. However, these contractions do not culminate in labour: They occur at irregular intervals and there is no progressive increase in the frequency/intensity of these painful contractions. The pain is more like a discomfort in the lower abdomen and is not like true labour pain, which starts from back and radiates to the lower abdomen. False labour pains are not associated with cervical dilatation or show. The discomfort is relieved by sedation.

In those instances where the diagnosis of true labour is not established with certainty, the only way to identify false labour pain is to observe the woman for sometime: if the contractions go away without causing progressive dilatation and effacement of cervix with descent of head, we know that they were false pains.

True labour pains	*False labour pains*
Contractions occur at regular interval	Contractions occur at irregular interval
Intervals gradually shorten	Intervals remain long
Intensity gradually increases	Intensity remains unchanged
Pain starts from back and radiates to the lower abdomen	Pain/ discomfort is usually in the lower abdomen
Cervix dilates	Cervix does not dilate
Pains are not stopped by sedation	Pains are relieved by sedation

Q4. What are Braxton-Hicks contraction?

Braxton-Hicks contractions are irregular uterine contractions that are *painless*. From the first trimester onwards, these contractions appear unpredictably and sporadically and are usually nonrhythmic and have low intensity. Towards term, they become more frequent and may cause some lower abdominal discomforts but are not associated with any cervical change.

Q5. When a pregnant woman presents in labour, what all are to be examined?

Much of what is to be routinely examined in a patient in labour is already given in case 4A. They are recapitulated in Table 4.1.

Table 4.1: Examination of a labouring patient

Points to be examined	*Observations in case 4A*
General examinations:	
General status	GC fair
Pulse, BP, temperature	Pulse: 80/min, regular BP: 120/80 mmHg Temperature: afebrile (generally we check temp. only by touch, therefore febrile/ afebrile. If febrile to touch or any S/S/ high risk for infection then check temperature with thermometer)
Pallor	Mild
Any associated finding	No pedal oedema, chest and CVS: NAD
Abdominal examination:	
Fundal height	Uterus term size
Number of fetuses	Singleton fetus,
Lie	Longitudinal lie
Presentation	Cephalic
presenting part fixed or not	Fixed, cephalic 3/5th above brim
Amount of liquor	Adequate
Uterine contractions: Duration, frequency	Mild contractions present 20 sec/5 min
Fetal heart rate (post contraction)	FHS +nt, 140/min, regular
Pelvic examination:	
Cervix: Dilatation (in cm), effacement	P/V: Cervix 2.5 cm dilated, 75% effaced
Status of membranes: (If ruptured: color of liquor)	membranes intact
Presenting part (in cephalic presentation: vertex/ brow/face	Vertex
Position of the presenting part in relation to maternal pelvis (e.g. left occipitoanterior)	LOA position
Station of presenting part (descent) in relation to ischial spines	Vx at -2 station
Pelvic assessment: Whether pelvis is adequate for delivery of the fetus; whether there is cephalopelvic disproportion	Pelvis adequate

Q6. If the fetus is big, the pelvis will appear to be contracted. Is not the term 'contracted' pelvis, therefore, a relative term?

The term cephalopelvic disproportion (CPD) is indeed a relative term. The term contracted pelvis is used only for a gross contraction that will not allow any fetus to deliver.

Q7. How do you clinically diagnose contracted pelvis/cephalopelvic disproportion?

In cephalic presentation, we feel, per abdominally, the level of head above the pelvic brim.

1. If the head is 0/5th or 1/5th above the brim, i.e. if it has entered the brim, it indicates that there is no inlet contraction.
2. If head is 5/5th or 4/5th above the brim, i.e. if it is free, then with left hand we try to push the head inside pelvic inlet (brim). Simultaneously, the index and middle fingers of right hand are placed over the head just above pubic symphysis to mark position of head in relation to the pubic bones. In case of disproportion there is overriding of head over pubic symphysis.

3. If head is 2/5th to 3/5th above the brim, it rules out inlet contraction to some extent, and observation during labour will determine the adequacy of pelvis.

P/V examination allows a more accurate pelvic assessment. If it is a gynecoid pelvis, the station of presenting part can tell us about CPD. If head is at 0 station, it indicates adequacy of inlet. If head is at –1, –2, –3 station, then feel the sacral promontory, sacral curve, side walls of the pelvis, sacrosciatic notches, ischial spines, moblilty of coccyx, subpubic angle and transverse diameter of the outlet (TDO). In a gynecoid pelvis, the sacral promontory is not normally felt, sacral curve is generous, sidewalls are parallel, sacrosciatic notches admit two fingers, ischial spines are not prominent, inter-ischial spinous diameter does not allow the two fingers to touch B/L ISP at the same time, subpubic angle admits two fingers and TDO admits 4 knuckles.

To look for CPD we hold the head per abdominally with left hand and try to push it inside pelvic brim along the axis of inlet. Simultaneously, with the fingers of the other hand are inserted into the vagina to feel the station of the head in relation with ischial spines and see whether head is able to negotiate the inlet or not. When BPD passes through pelvic inlet, station of head is at 0, i.e. level of ischial spines.

Interspinous diameter, sacrosiatic notches and pelvic sidewalls tell us about midpelvis while TDO, subpubic angle and mobile coccyx depict the adequacy of pelvic outlet.

Q8. If the pelvis seems adequate initially, what are the findings that suggest CPD during monitoring in labour?

During course of labour, a CPD is suspected if:

- The progress of labour is slow (evident from partograph)
- The presenting part (usually the head) does not descend progressively despite good uterine contractions
- Caput formation and moulding (grade 2 or more) are detected on P/V examination
- FHR abnormalities and/or meconium in liquor indicate fetal distress.

Q9. What does rupture of membranes (amniotic sac) signify?

Membranes usually rupture spontaneously in advanced first stage of labour or at the onset of second stage of labour. If membranes rupture before onset of labour pains and if labour pains start within next hour, it is still considered as a normal labour. However, if the labour does not start within an hour of membrane rupture, it is known as premature rupture of membranes (PROM). If PROM occurs in preterm fetus (gestation <37 weeks) this is known as preterm PROM.

After rupture of membranes, the amniotic fluid leaks through the vagina and the amount of liquor around the fetus decreases. Rupture of membranes is significant for three reasons:

1. If presenting part is not fixed in the pelvis, the possibility of umbilical cord prolapse and cord compression is greatly increased.
2. Labour is likely to begin soon if the pregnancy is at or near term.
3. If delivery is delayed 24 hours or more after membrane rupture, intrauterine infection is more likely.

When the membranes are ruptured artificially, it is known as artificial rupture of membranes (ARM). It is a method of induction and augmentation of labour.

Q10. How do you monitor normal labour during the first stage of labour?

Once first detailed examination has been performed and decision for vaginal delivery labour is taken, labour is monitored in labour room. During labour monitoring, the following aspects need to be monitored and charted on partograph.

Maternal condition

- Hydration status
- Half-hourly pulse rate, BP and temp.
- 4 hourly urinary output

Fetal condition:

- Half-hourly fetal heart rate (immediate post contraction)
- Color of liquor after membranes rupture (every 30 min by vulval pad inspection)

Progress of labour:

- Duration and frequency of uterine contractions (every 30 min)
- Station of head by abdominal examination as 5th above brim every 1 hour
- Pelvic examination (every 4 hours if progress is satisfactory):
  - Cervical dilatation and effacement
  - Station of presenting part
  - Any caput, moulding
  - Liquor color

In a *normal labour*, maternal and fetal condition remain normal, no evidence of any distress is seen, uterine contractions increase progressively and then optimal contractions (3 in 10 min with contractions lasting >40 secs) continue till delivery, head descends down progressively as evident from abdominal and pelvis examination, only small caput and grade 1 moulding may be there and liquor remains clear.

Q11. Why is it necessary to monitor the fetal heart rate during labour?

Labour is stressful for the fetus. During uterine contractions, the blood supply to the fetus decreases and fetal distress may occur which, if unattended immediately, can cause fetal injury or fetal death. Fetal heart rate monitoring is the commonest way to monitor for fetal distress in labour. In low risk cases, fetal heart rate should be noted every 30 min in first stage and every 5 min in second stage. The ideal time to auscultate is the immediate post-contraction period. In high risk pregnancies, the FHR is monitored every 15 min in first stage and after every contraction in second stage. If fetal distress is suspected during the first stage of labour, fetal scalp blood pH is tested for confirmation. A small nick is given on the scalp and the blood flowing out is withdrawn in a capillary tube. In distressed fetus, the pH is <7.25. Fetal scalp blood sampling is not done routinely in our labour room.

Q12. What is the use of a partogram?

Due to the uniform pattern of recording all maternal and fetal events of labour on a single chart, the partogram makes it is easy to communicate the details of the case to the next team in labour room. This is important because all over the world, labour rooms are managed in shift duties.

The partogram contains preplotted alert and action lines which indicate the imminent course of labour (Fig. 4.1). The alert line starts at 4 cm dilatation with a slope of 1cm dilatation/ hour, which the minimum rate of cervical dilatation in normal labour during active phase. The *action line* is parallel and 4 hours to the right of alert line.

As soon as the *cervical dilatation graph* crosses to the right of the *alert line*, the doctors at peripheral health centers should shift the patient to a centre with emergency obstetric services and operative facilities before the graph touches the action line. When graph shifts to the right of the *action line*, it warrants some immediate action like augmentation with oxytocin or cesarean section.

Q13. How do you know that the patient has entered the second stage?

When the patient enters the second stage of labour, she starts complaining of very severe

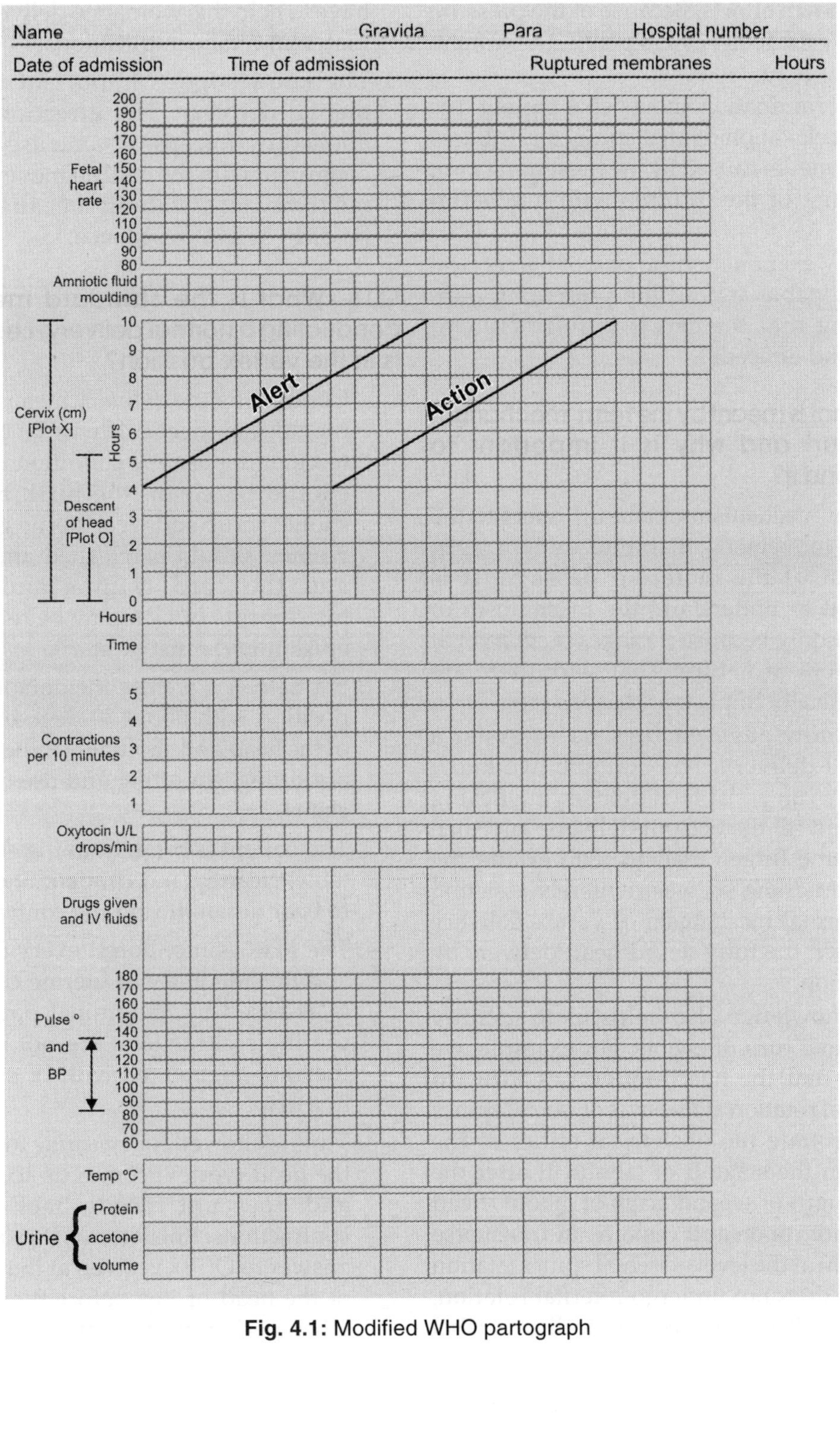

Fig. 4.1: Modified WHO partograph

pains. The contractions are associated with bearing down efforts. Because of the pressure exerted by the fetal head in pelvis, thc woman feels an urge to defaecate.

Local examination shows anal gaping due to reflex relaxation of anal sphincter, fullness in the perineum caused by the presenting part, and gaping of the inroitus with fetal scalp hairs.

On P/V examination, no part of the cervical rim is palpable around the presenting part, indicating that the cervix is fully (10 cm) dilated and effaced.

Q14. What is meant by the term 'mechanism of labour' and why is it important to understand it?

The term 'mechanism of labour' refers to the different movements that fetus undergoes to come out of the maternal passage. It is important to understand the mechanism of labour, if only because it makes us marvel at the wisdom of nature! That said, there are other clinically important reasons too:

1. The knowledge enables us to assist a normal delivery. For example, we know that we can assist fetal delivery by flexing the head till the occiput delivers, and then doing the Ritgen maneuvre to extend the head. In doing so, we are merely assisting the normal mechanism of vertex delivery in which the fully flexed head delivers by extension.
2. The knowledge also helps us to identify abnormal turn of events. For example, we know that the head undergoes forward internal rotation at the level of ischial spines to negotiate the obstetrical outlet of the fetus in the stage-II of labour. If after the full length of second stage of labour, head does not rotate and remains in transverse position at the level of ischial spines (station 0) and does not undergo internal rotation, labour will get arrested. Clinically, we label it as deep transverse arrest (DTA) and we have to help this woman to deliver to avoid maternal-fetal complications.
3. The knowledge is important in instrumental delivery. The direction of force applied by forceps or ventouse has to be congruent with the natural movements, i.e. mechanism of labour because that is passage of least resistance.

Q15. What is the standard method of conducting a normal delivery, i.e. the fetus is in the vertex position?

1. Conducting the delivery means assisting the normal mechanism of labour. It has to be under aseptic conditions: the table should be clean, the birth attendant should scrub and wear sterile gloves, the woman should be cleaned and draped, and the cord clamps and cutting instruments (which may be required for episiotomy) must be sterile.
2. For delivery, we use the dorsolithotomy position with about 30 degree elevation of the head and shoulders (others options are sitting, squatting and use of birthing chair).
3. The patient is brought to the edge of the table, cleaned and draped. She is asked to bear down during the contraction.
4. The FHR is monitored every 5 minutes and the adequacy of uterine contraction is assessed by abdominal palpation. If uterine contractions are not adequate, they are augmented with IV syntocinon in a drip.
5. Time is allowed for *crowning* to occur, i.e. the head (vertex) comes up to the vulva and does not recede back between contractions. Episiotomy, if required (*see* answer to Q.18), is given at the crowning of the head or just before the crowning when perineum is thinned out.

6. The perineum is supported with the left hand using a pad, and simultaneously the head is kept flexed with the right hand till the occiput is delivered. Thereafter, with the left hand, forward pressure is exerted on the fetal chin through the perineum just in front of the coccyx to assist extension of fetal head. This is called the *Ritdgen maneuver* which allows controlled delivery of the fetal head. Thereafter, the head extends, rotates laterally and delivers automatically. At this stage, care has to be taken that the cord does not loop around the neck.
7. After the head has delivered, check around neck for any loop of cord. If loop of cord is present, take measures to avoid stretching of cord during delivery (*see* answer to Q. 19). Hold the baby's head and try to assist the delivery of the shoulder. First the posterior shoulder, then the anterior shoulder and then the whole body comes out. The whole process takes only a few seconds.
8. Immediately after the baby comes, it is held upside down holding by its feet. The cord should be at or below the level of the delivery table so that no blood flows back from the baby to the placenta.
9. Once the baby is out, the newborn is placed at or below the level of the vaginal introitus for 30 seconds to 1 minute till no more blood comes from the placenta and the pulsations have almost disappeared. The cord is then clamped and cut, and the baby is handed over to the mother. Ideally, the baby should be put over the mother's abdomen so that mother can have a feel of the baby.
10. Immediately after delivery of the baby, the mother is given injection oxytocin 10 mg IM (alternatives: inj methergin 2 mg IV or misoprostol 600 mg orally/sublingually/rectally) to reduce blood loss in the third stage and prevent postpartum hemorrhage.
11. Time is allowed for the placenta to separate. The *signs of placental separation* are as follows:
    a. Uterus becomes globular and firmer
    b. Sudden gush of blood
    c. Uterus rises in the abdomen, because the placenta, having separated, passes down into the lower uterine segment and vagina, where its bulk pushes the uterus upward.
    d. Apparent lengthening of the umbilical cord.
12. After the placenta separates, it is delivered by controlled cord traction during uterine contraction with simultaneous counter-traction applied to the uterus with other hand. The placenta and membranes are checked for completeness. The uterus is massaged every 15 min for 1 hour to keep it contracted.

Q16. You have talked about assisting a delivery. About what percentage of delivery would fail without assistance?

If left to nature majority of labours will end in deliveries of the babies except for cases of obstructed labour, dysfunctional labour and rupture uterus. But if delivered without assistance, there will be more fetal and maternal complications like perineal/vaginal/periurethral tears, anal injuries, fetal injuries, fetal distress, fetal death (if tight cord around neck is there), fetal aspiration, shoulder dystocia, prolonged third stage with more blood loss, retained placenta, PPH, etc. Assistance during second stage of delivery is required to deliver baby without undue maternal and fetal complications.

Q17. Is there a need to give fundal pressure during labour?

No, fundal pressure should never be applied. It does not help at all; rather, it can cause inversion and rupture of uterus. Untrained *dais* often apply fundal pressure when the mother is exhausted and cannot bear down.

Q18. Is episiotomy routinely required? Does it require local anesthesia?

Episiotomy should be done only if perineal stretching is inadequate so that there is no perineal tear during delivery. A surgical wound heals better than a perineal tear. It is not required if the perineum is relaxed and stretches adequately, which is usually so in multiparous women.

Episiotomy should never be done without local anesthesia. It should be stitched properly after delivery. After it is stitched, the episiotomy site must be continuously observed for hematoma until the patient is shifted to the postnatal ward. Sometimes there is a bleeder in the episiotomy causing a huge bulge in the vulva or a collection in the vagina that compresses the urethra so that the patient is unable to pass urine. Occasionally, blood transfusion may be required.

Episiotomy is required in majority of the cases of forceps delivery as for introduction of forceps blade inside vagina more space is required. Only in cases of very lax perineum episiotomy may not be required.

Q19. What should be done if the cord loops around the neck of the baby during delivery?

If it is a loose cord, it can be slipped over the head so that it does not get tightened or stretched when the baby comes out. *If it is a tight cord,* it is clamped at two places and cut in between so that the cord get disentangled from the neck, before delivering the shoulders and body of the fetus. Cutting the cord a little too early does not harm the baby if its head is out.

Q20. Is instrumental delivery synonymous with forceps delivery?

No, it can also be a ventouse delivery. In Ventouse delivery, a suction cup that is applied to the head near the occiput and a vacuum is created in the cup over a period of 8 minutes. The suction pulls the scalp, creating a *chignon* on the head that fits nicely into the cup. The baby can now be pulled out by pulling on the suction cup. The advantage of ventouse is that it can be applied even when the cervix is not fully dilated and the head is not fully rotated.

Q21. Has ventouse replaced the forceps?

No, both have their own advantages. Delivery is rapid with forceps and slower with ventouse. If the cervix is fully dilated, and head has well descended then you can apply forceps and take out the baby within a minute. Moreover, we avoid vacuum in preterm deliveries since putting it on the fetal scalp injures it. Also, we cannot apply ventouse on breech and face.

Q22. After delivery of the head, is it necessary to wipe out the nose or mouth in the process of delivery?

Once the thorax is delivered, newborn can aspire and there may be aspiration of amniotic fluid, particulate matter and blood whatever is in contact with fetal face. To prevent this aspiration, face is quickly wiped and mouth suction is advocated to aspirate the nares and mouth when the head comes out.

Q23. Babies have been born for millions of years. Why is it important today to cut the cord?

We can keep the baby with the cord and let the placenta deliver but then it will delay the handing over of the baby to pediatrician. Half an hour is the duration of the third stage and we have to wait for placental separation. Moreover, we nowadays promote active management of third stage of labour as it helps in preventing postpartum hemorrhage. Therefore we prefer to cut the cord and proceed rather than waiting for nature to take its course.

Q24. Does the baby have to be resuscitated?

Ten percent of the babies require resuscitation to stimulate breathing. Also if there is meconium stained liquor, it is important to immediately do suction to prevent aspiration. Another important aspect is maintenance of temperature to prevent hypothermia. These basic steps are recommended for all deliveries.

Q25. What is Apgar score?

The score gives objective assessment of the condition of the newborn at birth. In cases of intrapartum fetal asphyxia or hypoxia, apgar scores at 1 min will be low. The 1 minute apgar score reflects the need for immediate resuscitation. The 5 minute apgar score is a useful index of the effectiveness of resuscitative efforts. The 5 minute apgar score also has prognostic significance for neonatal survival. Low apgar score of 0–3 for longer than 5 minutes correlates with adverse future neurological outcomes.

Table 4.2: Apgar score

	0	*1*	*2*
Respiration	Nil	Slow	Crying
Heart rate	Nil	<100	>100
Tone	Flaccid	In between	Flexed
Reflex response	Nil	Grimace	Cry
Color	Pale or blue	Peripheral cyanosis	Pink

Q26. In the middle of the night in a residential colony, a woman has labour pains and the next-door MBBS doctor is summoned. Should (s)he try to assess the labour pains as true or false, or advise immediate shifting to a maternity clinic?

The doctor should assess whether the woman has true or false labour pains or if she merely has abdominal colics. (S)he should also look for signs like the 'show' and rupture of membranes. (S)he must listen to the fetal heart sound to look for signs of fetal distress. If these suggest labour then she should be shifted to the maternity centre. It is better to err and send a woman who is not in labour to the hospital than not sending a woman in labour to the hospital.

Q27. How is a normal vaginal delivery done at home or in a rural area?

Home delivery is not difficult. Five C's are important to be taken care of by the birth attendants, i.e. clean surface, clean hand, clean cut, clean cord tie and clean cord stump. Such deliveries are conducted by traditional birth attendants. WHO recommends that all deliveries should be conducted by skilled birth attendants. A skilled birth attendant is an accredited health professional–such as midwife, doctor or nurse–who has been educated and trained to proficiency in the skills needed to manage normal (uncomplicated) pregnancies, child birth and the immediate postnatal period, and in the identification, management and referral of complications in women and newborns.

Delivery kits are provided to the birth attendants The kit contains clean cloth, sterile blade to cut cord and clean thread to tie cord. If the kits are not available, they can be prepared during antenatal period in advance of the labour. A useful drug for deliveries at periphery is misoprostol 400–600 μg given oral or per rectal immediately after delivery to prevent PPH.

Q28. What should an MBBS doctor do if a woman in labour comes to the hospital with some complication, say, a partially-delivered leg of a breech baby?

The management will depend on several factors:

i. The period of gestation
ii. Fetal heart sound
iii. Cervical dilatation
iv. Pelvis adequacy

Assessment	Management
Alive baby, term pregnancy, cervix fully dilated, pelvis adequate	Assisted vaginal breech delivery
Alive baby, term pregnancy, primi with undilated cervix or inadequate pelvis	Preferably cesarean section
Alive baby, term pregnancy, multi with undilated cervix, adequate pelvis	Observe labour till full cervical dilatation, deliver by assisted vaginal breech delivery
Preterm baby with leg hanging out with partially dilated cervix	If baby is salvageable, do an LSCS, if baby is not salvageable because of extreme prematurity, wait for vaginal delivery.
FHS absent	Wait for vaginal delivery

The role of an MBBS doctor first attending such patient in labour is to immediately assess the patient regarding above parameters so that a plan of management can be formed as one of the following:

1. Immediate cesarean section
2. Assisted vaginal delivery
3. Monitoring of labour till second stage for Assisted vaginal delivery.

He/she should call the senior most obstetrician available in labour room to conduct the breech delivery or to assess, counsel and finalise the mode of delivery.

Q29. What are the problems encountered during delivery?

Different complications can occur in different stages of labour and these can be maternal or fetal complications. Both low and high risk labours need to be monitored closely. The complications that can occur are:

Fetal distress: Signs of fetal distress are *FHR abnormalities* (fetal bradycardia, fetal heart decelerations with contractions) and *meconeum stained liquor*. Fetal distress can be confirmed by detection of acidosis on fetal scalp blood pH.

If fetal distress is detected in second stage of labour, immediate instrumental delivery is done. If fetal distress is detected in the first stage of labour, oxytocin (if on flow) is stopped, the patient is turned to the left lateral position and given oxygen. If fetal distress persists and delivery is not imminent, a cesarean section is done. If vaginal delivery is imminent, it is allowed to continue. If there is only meconeum staining, an amnioinfusion can be done.

Cord accidents: Cord prolapse can occur in malpresentations in labour or if membranes rupture while head is free floating. If cord prolapse occurs immediate delivery (vaginal or cesarean section depending on cervical dilatation) is required to save the baby.

Fetal death: Fetal death can occur if above two are not urgently managed. Fetal death can occur in cord accidents if true cord knot is there or multiple cord loops around fetal neck are there. Fetal death can also occur in the event of massive abruption, cord compression in cases with severe oligohydramnios, severe IUGR, abnormal fetus.

Fetal injuries during delivery: If the baby is big, there can be shoulder dystocia and difficulty in delivering the shoulders. In breech delivery, there can be difficulty and fetal injuries during the delivery of the baby.

Abnormal progress of labour: Early detection of slow labour progress is necessary for preventing fetal distress and maternal exhaustion.

The ***first stage of labour*** (cervical dilatation or descent of the presenting part) can be prolonged due to CPD or inefficient/discordant uterine contractions. The prolongation is readily apparent if the labour is charted on a partograph. If the contractions are mild, they are augmented with oxytocin provided there is no CPD. If there is CPD, a Cesarean delivery is done.

If the ***second stage of labour*** is prolonged (Primi >2 hours; Multi >1 hour), assess maternal hydration, fetal condition, uterine contractions, pelvis adequacy and rotation of head. If the uterine contractions are strong and there are no contraindications, an instrumental delivery is conducted.

Maternal complications: Prolonged labour causes maternal exhaustion which is characterized by dehydration, tachycardia, and fever. Rupture uterus can result because of previous uterine scar, mismanaged prolonged labour or inadvertant use of oxytocics. Hemorrhage can occur due to placenta previa or abruption, and patients with severe anemia or heart disease can go into shock.

Third stage complications: Postpartum hemorrhage (atonic and traumatic) can occur before or after delivery of the placenta. PPH is a life threatening complication and a major cause of maternal mortality. Hence, for one hour after delivery, the woman should be closely monitored for bleeding. Another complication that can occur during delivery of the placenta is uterine inversion. This occurs if placenta is pulled while uterus is relaxed or counter traction to the uterus is not applied.

Q30. Why is it important to check whether placenta has been expelled or not in a case of PPH?

The mean time from delivery until placental expulsion is eight to nine minutes. Longer intervals are associated with an increased risk of postpartum hemorrhage, with rates doubling after 10 minutes. If PPH occurs in a case while placenta is still inside, manual removal of placenta has to be done under anaesthesia along with other resuscitative measures.

Q31. How long after a normal vaginal delivery should the mother start walking?

She should start walking about as soon as possible, go to the toilet when necessary and rest when she needs to. She may prefer to stay in bed for the first 24 hours or longer if she has an extensive perineal repair.

Q32. When should the breastfeeding start after delivery?

Breastfeeding should ideally be initiated within half an hour of a normal delivery (or within two hours of a caesarean section, or as soon as the mother regains consciousness).

Q33. What advice is given to the mother regarding breastfeeding?

Breastfeeding should be exclusive feeding to the child for first 6 months. It should be Demand feeding: Feed the baby whenever he/she demands (cries) for it. Complementary feeding should be started after 6 months.

Q34. Should the baby be kept separate from the mother?

No, the mother and baby should be kept in the same room and preferably on the same bed. This practice is known as "rooming in". This practice should be encouraged as it has certain advantages. First, it makes demand feeding easier to practise, as the mother can hear the child cry. Second, it keeps the baby warm, thus preventing hypothermia in the newborn. Third, it helps build a bond between the mother and the baby.

Q35. How long do you keep a woman in the hospital after a normal vaginal delivery?

We keep the patient in the labour room during the 4th stage and 3–4 hours after that. When she has passed urine, we shift the patient from the labour room to the postnatal ward. Early ambulation is important.

Although we can discharge the patient as early as 6 hours, in an institutional delivery, we would like to observe the baby too. If the patient has had normal delivery and the baby has accepted the feed for 24 hours and has passed urine and stools, the patient is discharged. Therefore, it usually takes about 24 hours for the patient to be discharged from the hospital.

LABOUR ROOM MINOR PROCEDURES

Assessment of Cervical Ripening

Before inducing labour, it is important to examine and assess the condition of the cervix, and assign it a score based on the criteria listed in Table 4.3 (Bishop Score):

- If the score is ≥6, the state of the cervix is favourable for labour, which is usually successfully induced with oxytocin alone.
- If the score is <6, the state of the cervix is unfavourable for labour and it needs to be ripened using prostaglandins or a Foley catheter before induction.

Preinduction Ripening of the Cervix

Prostaglandins are highly effective in ripening the cervix. Prostaglandin E_2 (PGE_2 or dinoprostone) is available in gel form in a 2.5 ml syringe that contains 0.5 mg of dinoprostone. PGE_2 gel is inserted intracervically and cervix is reassessed after 6 hours. If the cervix is still not ripe, the same dose can be reinserted upto a maximum of three doses. Alternatively, PGE_1 tablet (misoprostol) 25 μg tablet is placed in the posterior fornix of the vagina, and repeat after 4–6 hours. If there is no response after two doses of 25 μg, the dose is increased to 50 μg every 6 hours up to a maximum four doses (200 μg). Misoprostol is more effective in cervical ripening and labour induction but is associated with greater chances of uterine hyperstimulation and fetal distress. In all women undergoing ripening of cervix with prostaglandins, the uterine contractions and fetal heart rate are monitored for the first 2 hours

Table 4.3: Assessment of cervix for induction of labour

Factor	*Rating*			
	0	*1*	*2*	*3*
Dilatation (cm)	Closed	1–2	3–4	more than 5
effacement	0–30%	31–50%	51–80%	≥80%
*Consistency	Firm	Average	Soft	-
Position	Posterior	Mid	Anterior	-
Descent by station of head (cm from ischial spines)	–3	–2	–1, 0	+1, +2

*A firm cervix is like tip of nose while ripe cervix as soft as lips

Table 4.4: Oxytocin infusion rates for induction of labour (Note 1 mL = approximately 15 drops)

Time since Induction (hours)	*Dose (mIU/min)*	*Oxytocin concentration*	*Method of preparation*	*Drops/min*
0.00	2	4mIU/ml	2.0 units in 500 ml dextrose or normal saline*	8
0.30	4	4mIU/ml	Same	15
1.00	8	4mIU/ml	Same	30
1.30	16	4mIU/ml	Same	60
2.00	32	8 mIU/ml	4 units in 500 ml dextrose or normal saline	60
2.30	48	12 mIU/ml	6 units in 500 ml dextrose or normal saline	60
3.00	64	16 mIU/ml	8 units in 500 ml dextrose or normal saline	60

* 5% dextrose should be avoided as it being hypotonic solution can cause water retention and hyponatremia

Prostaglandins administration is discontinued and infusion of oxytocin is started if:

a. Cervical ripening has been achieved,
b. The membranes rupture,
c. Labour starts. Oxytocin induction is started at least 6 hours after PGE_2 gel administration or 4 hours of using misoprostol.

The *Foley catheter* (mechanical dilatation method) is an effective alternative where prostaglandins are contraindicated, e.g. previous caesarean or bronchial asthma. It should, however, be avoided in women with obvious cervicitis or vaginitis, a history of bleeding or ruptured membranes. The catheter is inserted into the uterus so that its inflatable bulb lies beyond the internal os. The bulb is inflated with 10 ml of water. The catheter is left in place till contractions begin and the catheter is expelled out. If nothing happens for up to 12 hours, remove the catheter and proceed with oxytocin.

Oxytocin Infusion

Oxytocin is given in infusion. In our hospital, we use the low dose protocol: It is started from 2 mIU/ml and doubled every 30 minutes depending on uterine contractions till 32 mIU/minute (Table 4.4). The dose of oxytocin is increased till the uterine contractions are adequate, i.e. three contractions in 10 minutes, each lasting for more than 40 seconds. This rate is maintained until delivery. The uterus should relax between contractions. Maximum dosage recommended is 42 mIU/min, but in primigravidas we sometimes use up to 64 mIU/min with caution. The dosage schedule in augmentation of labour is similar to that of labour induction.

Monitoring of the Patient on Oxytocin Drip

Oxytocin can hyperstimulate the uterus, causing fetal distress and, rarely, uterine rupture. One should watch for water intoxication. Multiparous women are at higher risk of uterine rupture. Hence, during oxytocin infusion, the maternal pulse, BP, urine output, uterine contractions and fetal heart should be charted every 30 minutes. FHS should be recorded at the end of an uterine contraction.

- If the fetal heart rate is less than 100 beats per minute, stop the infusion. Put the patient in left lateral position and start ringer lactate IV infusion and oxygen inhalation.

- If hyperstimulation occurs (i.e. any contraction lasts longer than 90 seconds, or if there are more than five contractions in 10 minutes), stop the infusion. Discontinuation of oxytocin infusion rapidly reduces its plasma concentration (with a half-life of approximately 5 minutes) and is associated with a rapid decrease in the frequency of contractions. If uterus does not relax then tocolytics (terbutaline 250 mcg subcutaneous) are given.

Contraindications for Oxytocin Infusion

Oxytocin infusion is contraindicated in conditions in which vaginal delivery is contraindicated, e.g. fetopelvic disproportion. Other contraindications include:

- Abnormal fetal presentation
- Marked uterine overdistension such as hydramnios, multiple fetuses, very large fetus
- High parity (Six or more)
- Previous uterine scar: In cases with previous one LSCS oxytocin can be given with caution
- Distressed fetus.

Artificial Rupture of Membranes (ARM)

ARM is done for induction or augmentation of labour. Membrane rupture, whether spontaneous or artificial, often sets off the following chain of events:

1. Expulsion of amniotic fluid;
2. Decrease in uterine volume;
3. Production of prostaglandins, stimulating labour; and
4. The appearance (if the woman is not in labour) or intensification (if she is already in labour) of uterine contractions.

Procedure

- Auscultate and record the fetal heart rate.
- Ask the woman to lie on her back with her legs bent, feet together and knees apart.
- Wearing gloves, use one hand to examine the cervix and note the consistency, position, effacement and dilatation.
- Use the other hand to insert a Kocher's clamp into the vagina.
- Guide the clamp towards the membranes along the fingers in the vagina.
- Place two fingers against the membranes and gently rupture the membranes with the instrument in the other hand. Allow the amniotic fluid to drain slowly around the fingers.
- Note the colour of the fluid (clear, greenish, bloody). If thick meconium is present, suspect fetal distress.
- After ARM, listen to the fetal heart rate during and after a contraction. If the fetal heart rate is abnormal (less than 100 or more than 180 beats per minute), suspect fetal distress.
- If good labour is not established 1 hour after ARM, begin oxytocin infusion.
- If labour is induced because of severe maternal disease (e.g. sepsis or eclampsia), begin oxytocin infusion at the same time as ARM.

Precautions

- In hydramnios, sudden decrease in intra-amniotic pressure can result in separation of placenta (abruption placentae), therefore one must do controlled ARM in these cases.
- In cases of free head, there is a possibility of cord prolapse after ARM. Therefore ARM should be done only once head is fixed.

Therefore, after every ARM procedure listen to FHS and look for bleeding P/V.

Episiotomy

Indications

Episiotomy is not to be done indiscriminately in all cases of primigravidas, as was practiced earlier. It is to be performed in cases with rigid perineum where tear is likely to occur if episiotomy is not performed, e.g. in the case of:

- Complicated vaginal delivery (breech, shoulder dystocia, face presentation, face to pubes presentation, forceps, vacuum delivery);
- Rigid perineum, scarring or poorly healed perineal tears.

Procedure

- Rule out known allergies to lignocaine or related drugs. Lignocaine can cause seizures and death that are more often due to accidental iv injection than due to allergy. Hence, aspirate (pull back on the plunger) to be sure that no vessel has been penetrated. If blood is aspirated into the syringe, pull out the syringe and try again. Never inject lignocaine if blood is aspirated. The maximum dose of lignocaine is 20 mg, i.e. 20 ml of 1% lignocaine solution.
- Anaesthetize early to provide sufficient time for effect. After cleaning and draping, and taking full aseptic precautions, infiltrate about 10 ml 0.5% lignocaine solution beneath the vaginal mucosa, beneath the skin of the perineum and deeply into the perineal muscle (Fig. 4.2). Wait for 2 minutes and then pinch the incision site with forceps. If the woman feels the pinch, wait for 2 more minutes and then retest.
- Performing an episiotomy will cause bleeding. It should not, therefore, be done too early. Wait to perform episiotomy until the perineum is thinned out and 3–4 cm of the baby's head is visible during a contraction: It should be done just before crowning and not at the crowning.
- Place two fingers between the baby's head and the perineum. Use scissors to cut the perineum about 3–4 cm in the mediolateral direction (Fig. 4.3). Use scissors to cut 2–3 cm up the middle of the posterior vagina. Carefully examine for extensions and other tears after delivery of the baby.

Repair of Episiotomy

- Absorbable sutures should be used for closure. Polyglycolic sutures (e.g. vicryl rapid) are preferred over chromic catgut for their tensile strength, non-allergenic

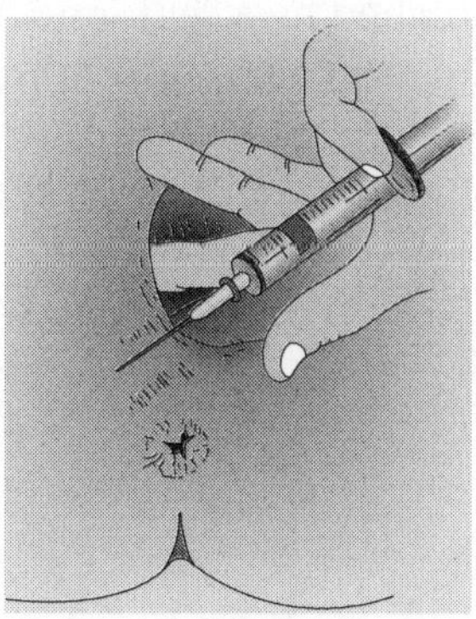

Fig. 4.2: Infiltration of perineal tissue with local anaesthetic

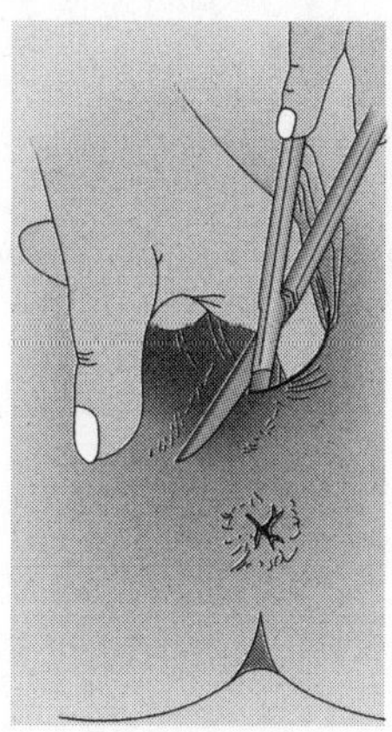

Fig. 4.3: Making the incision while inserting two fingers to protect the baby's head

properties and lower probability of infectious complications and episiotomy breakdown. Chromic catgut is an acceptable alternative, but is not ideal.

- If the episiotomy is extended through the anal sphincter or rectal mucosa which can be confirmed by per rectal examination, manage as third or fourth degree tears, respectively and a senior person should repair this.
- Episiotomy is stitched in 3 layers:
  - Close the vaginal mucosa using continuous 2–0 suture (Fig. 4.4A). Start the repair about 1 cm above the apex (top) of the episiotomy. Continue the suture to the level of the vaginal opening.
  - Close the perineal muscle using interrupted 2–0 sutures (Fig. 4.4B).
  - Close the skin using interrupted (or subcuticular) 2–0 sutures (Fig. 4.4C).

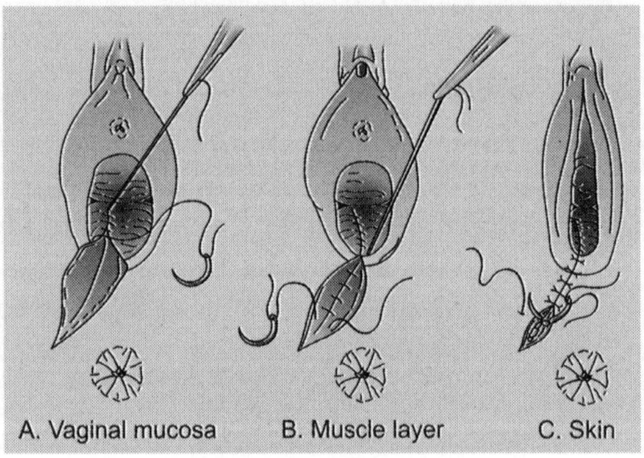

Figs 4.4A to C: Repair of episiotomy

Complication of Episiotomy

Episiotomy haematoma can occur in immediate post operative period, for which patient has to be resuscitated first and the haematoma is drained in operation theatre by opening the episiotomy sutures, holding the bleeder and restitching the episiotomy.

In late complications, there can be dehiscence of episiotomy wound (gaped episiotomy). For this local antiseptic douche is given and episiotomy is resutured once the margins of the wound are healthy.

Repair of Perineal Tears

There are four degrees of tears that can occur during delivery: *First degree tears* involve the vaginal mucosa and connective tissue. *Second degree tears* involve the vaginal mucosa, connective tissue and underlying muscles and skin (like episiotomy). *Third degree tears* involve complete transection of the anal sphincter. *Fourth degree tears* involve the rectal mucosa.

If the tear is long and deep through the perineum, inspect to be sure that there is no third or fourth degree tear: Place a gloved finger in the anus and gently lift the finger to identify the sphincter and feel its tone (tightness).

First and second degree perineal tear are stitched in the same way as an episiotomy is sutured. Third and fourth degree perineal tear should be stitched by a senior doctor in good light. Rectal mucosa, anal sphincter and perirectal fascia need to be stitched properly. Rest of the repair is same as for episiotomy.

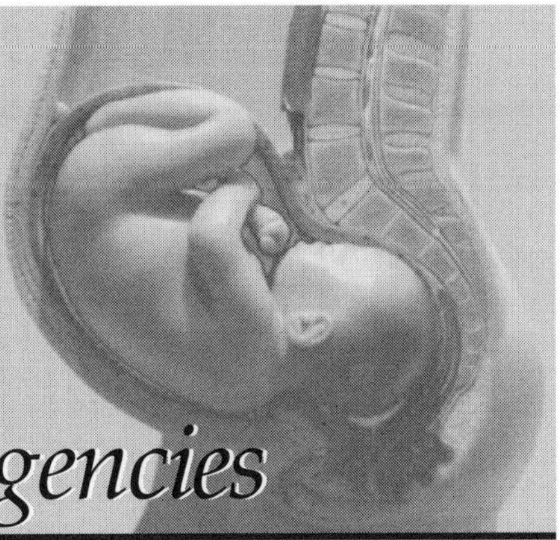

5 Obstetrical Emergencies

CASE 5A OBSTRUCTED LABOUR

A 18-year-old primigravida with 9 months amenorrhoea
C/o labour pains and leaking P/v for 2 days
C/o continuous pain abdomen since morning
Delivery was attempted by a *Dai* but was unsuccessful
C/o loss of fetal movements for 1 day

Pregnancy was unbooked and unsupervised
No significant history

O/E: Short statured, height: 130 cm
Dehydrated
Pallor +
Febrile, Temp: 100°F
Pulse: 120/min
BP: 110/80 mmHg
Chest/CVS: NAD

P/A: Uterus term size
Single fetus, cephalic 4/5th above brim
FHS not localized
Lower uterine segment stretched and tender
Upper segment retracted
Bandl's ring present

Q1. Why did you diagnose this patient as a case of obstructed labour?

The history of prolonged labour, failure to deliver, and the cessation of labour pains after 2 days of ineffective pains, and the general appearance of the patient (short statured, and dehydrated with tachycardia) are all suggestive of obstructed labour. The possibility is further strengthened following abdominal examination which shows that the widest diameter of the fetal head is felt above the pelvic brim (because it is unable to descend), the lower uterine segment is stretched, and the Bandl's ring is present. The absence of fetal movements and fetal heart sounds, indicating fetal death, are corroborative. On vaginal examination, the oedema of the vulva and cervix suggests that the woman has been bearing down for a long time. Dehydration made the vagina hot and dry. The diagnosis is clinched by a large caput succedaneum, an excessively moulded fetal head stuck in pelvis, and a contracted pelvis.

Q2. You have noted that Bandl's ring is present in the patient. What is Bandl's ring?

Bandl's ring is a late sign of obstructed labour. It is a horizontal line of depression across the

Uterus relaxed
L/E: Vulval oedema present
P/V: Vagina hot and dry
Cervix 6–7 cm with thick lips
Vertex at brim
Membranes absent
Caput +++
Moulding +++
No liquor obtained
Pelvis contracted at inlet and midpelvis
Diagnosis: Primigravida with term pregnancy with obstructed labour with intrauterine death

Adv:
Admit in emergency ward
Start I/V infusion with ringer lactate/normal saline
Inj antibiotics: Inj ampicillin 1 gm I/V AST, Inj gentamicin 80 mg I/V, metrogyl 400 mg I/V
Catheterise the bladder

Send investigations:
Hemoglobin, blood group, blood urea and serum electrolytes
Prepare for emergency cesarean section

Post operative special care
Prolonged catheterization for 7 days to prevent fistula formation.

abdomen at about the level of the umbilicus. The line delineates the grossly thickened, retracted upper uterine segment, and the dangerously thinned distended lower uterine segment. The lower abdomen is often further distended by a full bladder and gas in the intestines.

During normal pregnancy and labour, a constriction ring called *retraction ring* appears between the upper and lower uterine segments. Unlike the Bandl's ring, the retraction ring is not seen or felt per abdominally.

Q3. Why was the bladder catheterized in this case of obstructed labour?

The bladder was catheterised to prevent bladder injury. Post delivery, the catheter is kept in situ for 7–10 days to prevent vesico vaginal fistula formation as it helps in healing of ischemic tissues.

Q4. What can be the complications of obstructed labour if no action is taken?

If early action is not taken when signs of obstruction appear, it can lead to rupture uterus, genital fistulas (due to anoxic necrosis of bladder/vaginal/rectal tissues trapped between the fetal head and the pelvic bones), puerperal sepsis (due to early rupture of membranes), atonic PPH, DIC (due to sepsis or decay of the dead fetus), maternal mortality, fetal injury and death (due to excessive moulding which causes meningeal tear and intracerebral hemorrhage, or due to anoxia caused by pressure on the placenta and umbilical cord). Rupture of the uterus is more likely to occur in multipara (it is rare in nullipara), especially if the uterus is already weakened by the scar of a previous caesarean section. Rupture of the uterus causes haemorrhage and shock. The shock can also occur due to maternal dehydration. It is fatal without treatment. If the baby survives, it may have complications resulting from birth asphyxia, such as cerebral palsy and/or mental retardation.

Q5. Is 'obstructed labour' the same as 'prolonged labour'?

No. *Obstructed labour* means that, in spite of strong uterine contractions, the fetus cannot descend through the pelvis due to a problem with the ***P**assenger* (hydrocephalus, locked twins, or malpresentations), or with the ***P**assage* (contracted pelvis or tumour in the birth canal). CPD is the commonest cause of obstructed labour.

Prolonged labour occurs not only in obstructed labour but also when there is a problem with ***P**ower* (poor or uncoordinated uterine contractions). It is defined as the prolongation of labour (wherein labour is defined as the onset of regular, rhythmical painful contractions accompanied by cervical dilatation) beyond 24 hours. This definition, however, has limitations. It is more useful to specify which stage of labour is prolonged, e.g. "prolonged latent phase of labour" or "prolonged active phase of labour". In the normal course, the latent phase should not be longer than 8 hours, and the active phase should not last longer than 12 hours. Cervical dilatation is either slow or stops after a while.

Q6. Can an obstructed labour be avoided?

An obstructed labour can be avoided only through an early detection of prolonged labour (by use of partogram) and timely action (doing a caesarian section). The partogram plots the extent of cervical dilatation against time and therefore, it indicates the *rate* of cervical dilatation. If the partogram shows the cervical dilatation to be slow or slowing down, it portends a prolonged labour. Based on it, an early action can be taken without waiting for the full duration of the first stage. More vigilence is required in the case of teenage mothers: She has a greater chance of going into obstructed labour as her pelvis has not developed into its adult shape that allows the foetus to deliver normally.

Q7. Is prolonged labour harmful if there is no obstruction?

Excessively prolonged labours, even in the absence of any obstruction, may lead to maternal and/or fetal distress and is associated with a higher risk of infection due to increased intervention and frequent vaginal examinations.

CASE 5B RUPTURE UTERUS

A 30-year-old $G_2P_1L_0$ with 9 months amenorrhoea
H/o labour pains and leaking p/v for 1 days
c/o sudden severe pain abdomen with a feeling of something giving away in the abdomen 2 hours back with loss of fetal movements and bleeding p/v
C/o continuous pain abdomen since then.
Intermittent labour pains stopped
Patient fainted on way to hospital
Delivery was being conducted by dai at home

Pregnancy was unbooked and unsupervised
No significant history in antenatal period

Past obstetric history
Ist full term LSCS for prolonged labour in Pvt centre in a village 1 year back. Records NA
Baby died after 1 day

O/E: Short statured height: 130 cm
Dehydrated
Pallor +++
Afebrile
Pulse: 120/min
BP: 90/50 mmHg
Chest/CVS: NAD
P/A: Midline vertical infraumbilical scar present
Uterine contour not made out
Fetal parts felt superficially. Head high up
FHS not localized
A rounded firm mass felt in left upper abdomen adjoining the fetus.
L/E: Vulval oedema present
P/V: Vagina hot and dry
Cervix 2 fingers loose hanging

Q1. Which findings in this case suggest a ruptured uterus?

A rupture of uterus is suggested by bleeding p/v, and the sudden pain abdomen that is followed by a sudden cessation of labour pains. A h/o LSCS for prolonged labour (which could be an obstructed labour) is corroborative. General examination reveals shock. P/A examination reveals a lack of uterine contour and the superficiality of fetal parts. P/V examination reveals a loose hanging cervix and the absence of presenting parts.

Q2. Is another pregnancy possible or advisable after a rupture uterus?

Ideally pregnancy is not advisable after repair of rupture uterus as risk of recurrent rupture is very high. However, in cases like the present one where obstetric history is poor and the desire for subsequent pregnancy is very high, pregnancy can be allowed but only after 3 years or more, allowing the uterine scar to heal well. Being a high risk pregnancy, it should be well supervised in a tertiary care centre. Symptoms like pain abdomen and bleeding p/v during antenatal period should be taken seriously. The patient should be planned for elective cesarean section at 37 weeks. Ideally she should be hospitalized at 34 weeks and cesarean delivery should be undertaken before 37 weeks if she goes into labour or if a rupture uterus is suspected.

Q3. Why does the uterus rupture?

The uterus can rupture if the intrauterine pressure rises excessively, as in obstructed labour or following indiscriminate use of oxytocics (oxytocin and prostaglandins). It can also rupture if there is a weakness in the uterine wall, as in the case of a previous cesarean section, previous damage to myometrium due to myomectomy, D&C, manual removal of placenta, or uterine malformations. The uterus can also rupture due to trauma (traumatic rupture).

Q4. What procedure will be done during laparotomy?

Uterine rupture is a life threatening emergency. Depending on laparotomy findings procedure is decided. Aim is to stop the bleeding and reconstruct the uterus if feasible. Different procedures commonly done in a case of rupture uterus are:

- Hysterectomy
- Uterine repair with or without tubal ligation.

Generally in a case of rupture uterus with previous cesarean section, repair is possible. However, in obstructed labour rupture is huge and ragged making repair difficult. As this patient does not have any live issue, repair and preservation of the uterus will be tried if possible.

In a case of multipara with the live issues, we prefer to do either hysterectomy or tubal ligation with uterine repair as there is high risk of rupture in the next pregnancy. Conservative surgery (repair) is usually done in the following conditions:

- Low transverse rupture
- No extension to broad ligand, cervix or paracolpos
- Easily contollable hemorrhage
- Good general condition
- Desire for future childbearing
- No evidence of evolving coagulopathy.

Presenting part high up not felt with fingers

Fresh bleeding P/V on examination

Pelvis contracted at inlet and midpelvis

Clinical Δ: Rupture Uterus

Management:

Urgent Hb, Blood group, BT, CT, CRT, Urine Alb/sugar

Admit in emergency

I/V line and resuscitation with fluids

O_2 by mask

Catheterise the bladder

Injectable antibiotics

Arrange 3–4 units of cross-matched blood and start transfusion as soon as possible

Prepare for emergency laparotomy with consent for repair of uterus/hysterectomy as per operative findings

Investigations: Hemoglobin, serum electrolytes, bed side coagulation profile (BT, CT, CRT)

Postoperatively special care: Prolonged catheterization for 7–10 days

CASE 5C ATONIC POSTPARTUM HEMORRHAGE (PPH)

A 30-year-old P_2L_2
Delivered twins vaginally in labour room
30 minutes after delivery of placenta she started bleeding excessively
Pregnancy was supervised, antenatal period had no complications.
Pt admitted in active labour at 36 weeks
Duration of first stage 8 hrs, 2nd stage 1 hour, 3rd stage 20 min
Labour was uncomplicated.
Placenta was delivered after spontaneous separation. The placenta was examined and found to be complete.

O/E: Conscious and oriented
Pallor: ++
Pulse: 120/min, feeble
BP: 90/50 mmHg
RR: 24/min
Chest/ CVS: NAD
P/A: Uterus 24 weeks, soft and flabby
L/E: Bleeding from vagina ++
P/V: Vagina full of clots, removed
Cervical os open, clots present in uterus removed digitally

CI: Atonic PPH

Investigations
Hb with platelet count
Coagulation profile BT, CT, CRT
PT, PTTK

Management:
Call for help
Monitor BP and HR continuously
Start 2 I/V lines and give fast fluid

Q1. How much bleeding constitutes postpartum haemorrhage?

When >500 ml of blood is lost during delivery, it is called postpartum hemorrhage.

Q2. What are the usual causes of postpartum hemorrhage? What is the most probable cause in this patient?

The main causes of PPH are summarized by the 4 T's: Tone (atonia), trauma (genital trauma), tissue (retention of placental tissue) and Thrombin (bleeding diatheses). The patient was at high risk for atonic PPH as her uterus was overdistended due to multiple pregnancy. On examination, her uterus was found to be relaxed and therefore she is having atonic PPH.

Q3. What are the clinical signs of an atonic uterus?

The uterus is not well contracted and tends to relax after it is massaged. The bleeding is not continuous–it occurs in episodes, and the blood consists of dark red clots.

Q4. Can we predict and prevent PPH?

Risk factors are not identifiable in about 50% cases of atonic PPH. Hence, the possibility of PPH should always be kept in mind, since it causes haemorrhagic shock and is a major cause of maternal mortality. Anemic patients tolerate blood loss poorly and therefore antepartum correction of anemia is an important precaution. Active management should be done in all deliveries (active management described in chapter 4).

Q5. Why did you investigate for coagulation disorders?

Coagulation disorders, a rare cause of postpartum hemorrhage, are unlikely to respond to the measures described above. Therefore coagulation tests (at least the bedside tests like bleeding time, clotting time, clot retraction time) are done in all cases of PPH.

Q6. What are the complications of PPH?

PPH is major cause of maternal mortality due to haemorrhagic shock. Its complications include hypotension, anemia and fatigue, which may make maternal care of the newborn more difficult. Postpartum anemia increases the risk of postpartum depression. In the most severe cases, hemorrhagic shock may lead to anterior pituitary ischemia with delay or failure of lactation (i.e. postpartum pituitary necrosis or Sheehan's syndrome).

Q7. What are the drugs given if uterus is atonic?

Atonic uterus is treated with uterotonic agents, which include oxytocin, ergot alkaloids, and prostaglandins. *Oxytocin* is an effective first-line treatment for postpartum hemorrhage. It is administered either as 10 IU im, or 20–40 IU in 500 ml 5% glucose (125–250 ml/h). As much as 500 ml can be infused over 10 minutes without complications. *Methylergometrin* 0.2 mg im or iv, may be repeated as required at intervals of two to four hours. Because ergot alkaloid agents raise blood pressure, they are contraindicated in women with preclampsia or hypertension. *Prostaglandins* include $PGF_{2\alpha}$: Prostodin/Carboprost and PGE_1: Misoprostol. Carboprost can be administered intramyometrially or intramuscularly in a dose of 250 μg; this dose can be repeated every 15 minutes for a total dose of 2 mg. Hypersensitivity is the only absolute contraindication, but carboprost should be used with caution in patients with asthma or hypertension. Misoprostol can be administered sublingually, orally, vaginally, and rectally (1000 mcg).

Give injection Methergin 0.25 mg IV and start oxytocin infusion (20 units in 500 ml of saline and give at the rate of 60 drops/min)
If bleeding not controlled, give Inj Prostodin 250 μg I/M
Arrange and transfuse blood
Give oxygen by mask
Catheterise the bladder
Do uterine massage and bimanual uterine compression
Investigations: Hemoglobin with platelet count, coagulation profile
Side by side check for completeness of placenta removed and any genital tract tears
If bleeding not controlled with these measures, then take up for operative measures
Depending on patient's condition, as she is multiparous, early decision for hyster-ectomy can be taken up.

Q8. How do you perform bimanual uterine compression and massage?

Massage is performed by placing one hand in the vagina in anterior fornix and pushing against the body of the uterus while the other hand compresses the fundus from above through the abdominal wall. Posterior aspect of the uterus is massaged with the abdominal hand and the anterior aspect with the vaginal hand.

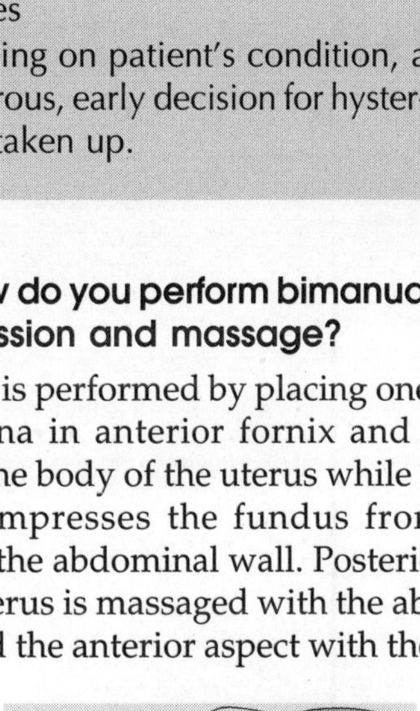

Fig. 5.1

Flow Chart 5.1: Algorithm for management of postpartum hemorrhage. Many of the steps involved in diagnosing and treating postpartum hemorrhage must be undertaken simultaneously. Although the steps in maternal resuscitation are consistent *(bold arrows)* other actions may differ based on the actual cause. (IV = intravenous; IU = international units; CBC = complete blood count; IM = intramuscularly; RBC = red blood cells; ICU = intensive care unit)

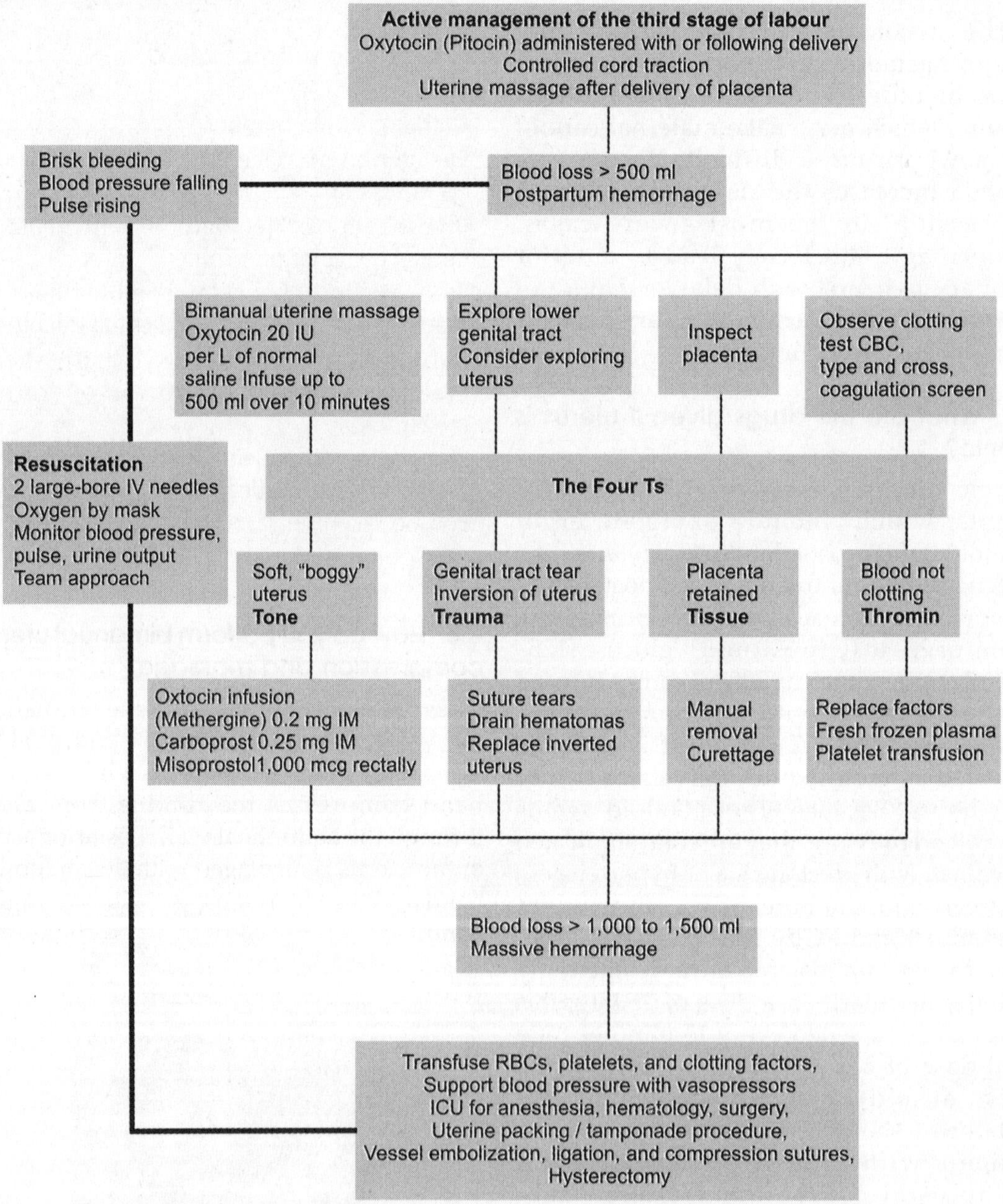

(Source: Am Fam Physician 2007;75:875-82)

Q9. If bleeding is not controlled with above means, what are other options?

If medical methods are unsuccessful, surgical management is required. If immediate surgery is not possible like delivery in primary centre or lack of expertise and patient has to be shifted to higher centre or sometimes when patient has coagulation disorder which need to be corrected before major surgery then following approaches can be utilized to stop bleeding from uterus and buy some time. Remember, these are not definitive measures.

Transvaginal uterine packing: About 8 to 10 M sterilized gauge is used to pack the uterine cavity from fundus to the cervix and total vaginal packing. Proper antibiotic coverage should be given.

Distended condom: A simple rubber catheter is put into condom and is doubly tied with a thread and is passed into uterine cavity and a tight pack is applied in the vagina with gauze. Condom is inflated with fluids by connecting catheter to the drip set. This causes uterine temponade and arrest bleeding. Other tubes which can be used are Sangstaken Blackmore tube or Foley's Catheter with a large bulb within the uterine cavity.

Q10. What are the surgical methods used in case of atonic PPH if needed?

Surgical approach can be radical (Hysterectomy) or conservative surgeries. Decision has to be taken depending on the patient's obstetric history, her general condition and surgeon's expertise.

Uterine Conservative Surgical Approach

Uterine compression suture: B-Lynch suture (Brace suture). It controls atonic PPH by providing an effective compression of the placental bed. This method is simple, effective and relatively safe life saving procedure.

Uterine artery ligation: The objective is to decrease blood flow to the uterus as about 90% of the uterine blood supply in pregnancy comes from these vessels. After ligation of uterine vessels if bleeding is not controlled, then the next step is to ligate the ovarian arteries.

Ovarian artery ligation: It arises directly from the abdominal aorta and anastomoses with uterine artery in the region of the uterine aspect of the utero-ovarian ligament. A suture is placed on the ovarian artery through avascular area in mesovarium. Procedure is repeated on the other side.

Bilateral internal iliac ligation-anterior division: The most important mechanism of action with internal iliac ligation is an 85% reduction in pulse pressure in those arteries distal to ligation, thus turning and arterial pressure system into one with pressure approaching those in venous circulation and leads to hemostasis via clot formation.

Angiographic arterial embolization: This is a new technique, conservative approach and offers a very high success rate. It is done by injecting gelatin particles through the internal iliac artery under radiological control. It offers temporary blockade. Various studies report a success rate of 75–100%.

Hysterectomy: It can be subtotal hysterectomy or total abdominal hysterectomy. The common indications are:

a. Abnormal placentation with placenta increta, acreta and percreta
b. Rupture uterus if tears are extensive and general condition of patient is poor.
c. Atonic PPH when other measures are not successful

CASE 5D PPH DUE TO GENITAL TRACT TRAUMA

A 24-year-old primigravida admitted at term pregnancy with labour pains

On admission her cervix was 4 cm dilated and fully effaced.
Uterine contractions good.
2 hrs later patient was bearing down
P/V examination revealed cervix to be 7 cm dilated and it was papery thin.

Within 20 min of her examination patient delivered while squatting on floor.
Cord was clamped and cut, baby handed over to pediatrician
Patient shifted to delivery table. Delivered placenta in 15 minutes.

1 hour after delivery patient sweating and restless
Continuous trickle of bright-red blood P/V.

On examination
Pallor ++
Pulse 110/min, feeble,
BP: 90/60 mmHg
P/A: Uterus was 20 weeks, well contracted
L/E: Fresh bleeding from vagina +

CI: PPH due to Genital Tract Trauma

Management:
Inv: Hb with platelet count, BT, CT, CRT (side by side with management)
2 I/V lines and fast fluids with oxytocin 20 units in one vac.
Oxygen by mask
Perspeculum examination to look for vaginal tear and cervical exploration followed by repair.

Q1. What is the most likely cause of the bleeding in this case, and why do you think so?

The most likely cause of bleeding in this case is a cervical tear because the patient delivered before full cervical dilatation. Note that the case sheet mentions: "P/V examination revealed cervix to be 7 cm dilated and it was paper-thin. Within 20 min of her examination patient delivered while squatting on floor."

Q2. You have mentioned 'cervical exploration' in management. What is cervical exploration?

Because cervix is very lax and loosely hanging, it is not possible to detect cervical tears by simple *per speculum* examination. For cervical exploration, the entire rim of the cervical lip is systematically examined in good light by applying two closely-spaced sponge-holding forceps on the cervical lip and stretching out the intervening segment, while an assistant retracts the vaginal walls anteroposteriorly using speculum and/or retractor. The bladder should be empty during the procedure.

Q3. How do you stitch the cervical tear?

When cervical tear is detected on exploration, both edges are held with the sponge holding forceps (as these are atraumatic and cervix is very vascular and friable during pregnancy). It is important to see the apex as sometimes the tear may be extending up in the lower uterine segment and thus requiring laparotomy for repair. If apex is easily visualized, then tear is stitched with first stitch applied just above the apex and rest of the tear is stitched with interrupted stitches using no. 1–0 vicryl or chromic catgut.

Q1. What is an inverted uterus?

The uterus is said to be inverted when its fundus descends and comes out of the cervix so that its inner surface becomes outer surface. The diagnosis of an inverted uterus must be considered if a patient without excessive vaginal bleeding suddenly goes into a shock during the third stage of labour. On abdominal examination, the uterus is not palpable. The uterus lies in the vagina or may even hang out of the vagina. There are four degrees of uterine inversion: 1st degree, in which the inverted fundus extends to, but not through the cervix. 2nd degree, in which the inverted fundus extends through the cervix but remains within the vagina. 3rd degree, in which the inverted fundus extends outside the vagina. *Total inversion*, in which both the vagina and the uterus are inverted.

Q2. What are the classical symptoms of uterine inversion?

Acute inversion presents most often with the triad of

1. Postpartum haemorrhage,
2. Sudden appearance of a vaginal mass, and
3. Shock. The sudden appearance of a large dark red mass accompanying the placenta is alarming. The pain is excruciating. The diagnosis is usually immediately obvious and is confirmed if the fundus cannot be palpated. Complete inversion is accompanied by severe shock, more than might be expected from the degree of blood loss alone.

Subacute and chronic cases are unusual and difficult to diagnose. They may present with spotting, discharge and low back pain. An USG may be required to confirm the diagnosis.

Q3. What are the causes of uterine inversion?

The commonest cause is excessive traction on the cord before placental separation. Hence it

CASE 5E INVERSION OF UTERUS

A 30-year-old P_4L_4 had vaginal delivery of live baby at home conducted by dai 1 hr back.

Placenta was delivered with difficulty.

Immediately after delivery of placenta a red mass appeared outside vagina

She had severe pain and had excessive bleeding

She became drowsy during transportation

O/E: Patient semiconscious

Dyspneic at rest

Radial pulse not palpable

BP not recordable

P/A: Uterus not palpable

L/E: Red mass seen coming out of the introitus. Whole vagina inverted out.

Clinical impression: Inversion uterus (fourth degree)

Management:

Admission in emergency

Start two IV lines and give fast fluids

Arrange and transfuse blood

Oxygen by mask

Catheterise the bladder

pethidine/diazepam IV

Cleanse inverted uterus using antiseptic solution

Apply compression to the inverted uterus with a moist, warm sterile towel until ready for the procedure

Reposit the inverted uterus in vagina if easily possible

No oxytocics till uterus is reposited back.

Prepare urgently for complete uterine reposition in pelvis under GA is important to apply controlled cord traction while simultaneously placing the other hand suprapubically, providing counter traction by pushing the uterus up. To prevent inversion, it is important never to pull on the cord without counter traction, never to pull it too hard and, if placenta does not descend, to wait till the next contraction. Application of fundal pressure during delivery, especially by untrained midwives, is a common cause of uterine inversion.

Q4. Does uterine inversion always present immediately after delivery?

No, uterine inversion may present acutely (within 24 hours of delivery), subacutely (over 24 hours and up to the 30th postpartum day), and chronic (more than 30 days after delivery). Very rarely, fundal submucous fibroid may cause chronic inversion uterus in nonobstetric cases.

Q5. What is the difference between repositioning in the vagina and repositioning in the pelvis?

Repositioning in vagina means that the inverted uterus pushed up into the vagina so that it does not hang outside. It is a temporary, incomplete measure that does not correct the inversion and does not require anesthesia. Complete repositioning in the pelvis involves correction of the inversion under general anesthesia.

Q6. How long after uterine inversion should one try to reposition it back?

In acute puerperal inversion, the uterus must be repositioned immediately. If immediate reposition is not possible, the uterus is at least repositioned in the vagina before preparing for a complete repositioning in the pelvis. If there is a long delay, a tight cervical ring forms around the inverted uterus that must be surgically incised to enable repositioning. In such cases it is prudent to wait for about 6 weeks to allow involution of the uterus before correcting the inversion surgically.

Q7. How is the uterus repositioned in the pelvis?

Repositioning of the uterus in the pelvis is done under general anesthesia. It can be done either hydrostatically or manually. Hydrostatic correction is much safer and should be tried first. The choice of the method also depends on the operator's experience and confidence. If both methods fail, repositioning is done under laparotomy by pulling the fundus up from abdomen while simultaneously pushing it up the vaginal. If the placenta is attached to the inverted uterus, it is removed only after correcting the inversion or at least when there is complete preparedness (including anesthesia) for correcting it.

For hydrostatic correction of uterine inversion, the woman is placed with her head lowered 0.5 metres below the level of the perineum (deep trendelenburg position), an IV drip set containing warm normal saline is placed 2 metres above the perineum, and a warm douche is started with the nozzle placed in the posterior fornix. The introital opening is obliterated with hand in vagina and arm wedging the introitus so that there is no leakage of fluid. The water distends the posterior fornix of the vagina gradually, increases the circumference of the orifice, relieves cervical constriction, and corrects the inversion.

Manual repositioning of the uterus is done by slowly pushing it up the vagina with the right hand. After reposition, methergin (0.25 mg IV stat) is given for inducing uterine contraction. The right hand is not removed immediately; instead, bimanual uterine compression and massage is continued till the uterus hardens and the bleeding stops. This is followed up with an oxytocin infusion (20 units in 500 ml of saline at 30–40 drops/min). Oxytocics and antibiotics are continued for at least 24 hours, and the patient is monitored closely to avoid reinversion.

If inversion occurs during delivery, it is repositioned immediately under IV sedation (diazepam or pethidine) only-general anesthesia is not required. If required, tocolytics (e.g. terbutaline 0.25 mg s/c) are administered to allow uterine relaxation.

Q8. If uterine inversion occurs with placenta still attached, how will the management differ?

Placenta is not removed till resuscitative measures have been started and preferably anaesthesia have been given in the OT and all is ready for reposition. Placenta is removed just before reposition.

CASE 5F ECLAMPSIA

A 20-year-old primigravida presented with amenorrhoea 36 weeks

C/o generalized tonic clonic convulsions 3 episodes in last 1 hour
H/o headache and vomiting before convulsions
H/o generalized swelling over body for 1 month

No h/o fever, epilepsy
HOPP: Unsupervised pregnancy
Past history: No h/o diabetes, epilepsy
O/E: Patient semiconscious, irritable
Responding only to painful stimuli
Pulse: 100/min, BP: 160/100 mmHg
RR: 24/min
Pallor: +, No icterus, cyanosis
Pedal oedema ++
Chest: Clear, CVS: NAD,
Neurological examination: NAD

P/A: Abdominal wall oedema +
Uterus 34 weeks, Single fetus in longitudinal lie, Cephalic presentation, Head 3/5th above brim, FHS 160/min, regular
Uterus irritable, neither tense nor tender

P/V: Cervix 2 cm dilated, 50% effaced, soft, central, Vertex at –2 station, membranes present, ARM done, clear liquor
Pelvis Adequate
Urine alb +++

Clinical diagnosis: Unbooked primigravida with 36 weeks pregnancy with antepartum eclampsia
Adv: Admit in gynae emergency: Eclampsia room
Secure airway
Do suction to remove secretions
O_2 by face mask SOS

Q1. What is eclampsia?

A pre-eclampsia complicated by generalized tonic clonic conulsions is termed as eclampsia. It is a pregnancy-specific multisystem disorder and convulsions are only one of the manifestations. Any convulsions during pregnancy are presumed to be eclampsia unless proved otherwise. The differentiating points are association with pre-eclampsia, onset >20 weeks of gestation, no previous history of epilepsy.

Q2. How would you manage a case of eclampsia?

The management of eclampsia involves six major steps:

1. Protection of airways and injury during convulsions,
2. Controlling the fits,
3. Controlling the BP,
4. Controlling the fluid balance,
5. Delivering the baby,
6. Giving care after delivery.

Respiratory care is achieved in four steps:

a. The woman is placed on her left side (in the semi-prone position) so that mucus or saliva can drain out;
b. The mouth and nostrils are cleaned by applying gentle suction and remove the secretions;
c. Oxygen is administered and continued for five minutes after each fit, or longer if cyanosis persists; and
d. Padded tongue blades or pads are placed between her teeth, which are secured to prevent aspiration.

The anticonvulsants given in eclampsia are magnesium sulphate (the drug of choice), phenytoin and diazepam. Inj $MgSO_4$ is continued till 24 hours after delivery or last fit whichever is later.

The goal of antihypertensive treatment is to keep the diastolic pressure between 90 and

100 mmHg to prevent cerebral haemorrhage. Oral Nifedipine/Hydralazine IV/Labetalol IV are given to control BP.

In all cases of eclampsia baby has to be delivered irrespective of the gestational age. Mode of delivery depends on fetal condition, cervical scoring and any contraindications to vaginal delivery. Aim during vaginal delivery is that baby should deliver within 12 hours of onset of eclampsia.

Q3. How is magnesium sulphate given?

For the loading dose, Inj. Magnesium sulphate 4 g (20 ml of 20% solution) is given slow IV, at the rate of 1 ml every minute. Thereafter, Inj. Magnesium sulphate is administered IM. Initially, 5 g should be injected into each gluteus muscle (10 ml of 50% solution, in each buttock), deep IM, with 1 ml of 2% Lignocaine in the same syringe.

If convulsions recur: An additional 2 g of Magnesium sulphate (10 ml of 20% solution) is given IV after 15 min. If the convulsions still continue, give diazepam.

After this 5 g of 50% $MgSO_4$ is given IM every 4 hours alternately in each buttock. Before giving the next dose of $MgSO_4$ we should ensure that: The urine output is at least 100 ml per 4 hours; Knee jerk reflexes are present; The RR is at least 16 breaths/minute.

Next dose is postponed if the above criteria are not met. If respiratory depression occurs (RR <16 breaths/minute) after giving $MgSO_4$, drug is discontinued. Antidote Calcium gluconate 1 g IV (10 ml of 10% solution) is given over a period of 10 minutes.

Q4. What complications can occur in eclampsia?

- Intracranial hemorrhage
- Pulmonary oedema due to aspiration pnemonitis or cardiac failure
- Blindness
- Hepatic rupture

I/V Line
Catheterise with Foley's catheter
Send Investigations
Fundus examination
Give Inj $MgSO_4$
Oral Depin 5 mg or Inj Labetalol 10 mg IV
Augment labour with syntocinon, and ARM
Vital monitoring, BP monitoring,
Intake/output charting
W/F progress of labour and FHS

- Liver failure
- Renal failure
- HELLP syndrome
- Disseminated intravascular coagulation
- Abruption
- Fetal distress
- Intrauterine death.

Q5. Is eclampsia a life-threatening condition?

Yes, the common causes of maternal mortality in eclampsia are:

1. Cerebral haemorrhage,
2. Pulmonary edema,
3. DIC and
4. Hepatorenal shutdown.

Q6. If a pregnant woman develops DIC, is it always due to eclampsia?

DIC in pregnancy has several causes and accordingly, the time of presentation varies. Commonly, it is seen in third trimester, during labour or postpartum. The commonest cause of DIC in pregnancy is placental abruption. Other causes are fetal death (if dead fetus is retained inside uterus for >4 weeks), amniotic fluid embolism (usually late stages of labour or immediate postpartum.), septicemia (puerperial sepsis and post-abortal sepsis) and abortion (septic abortion, intrauterine instillation of hypertonic saline or urea for second trimester abortions).

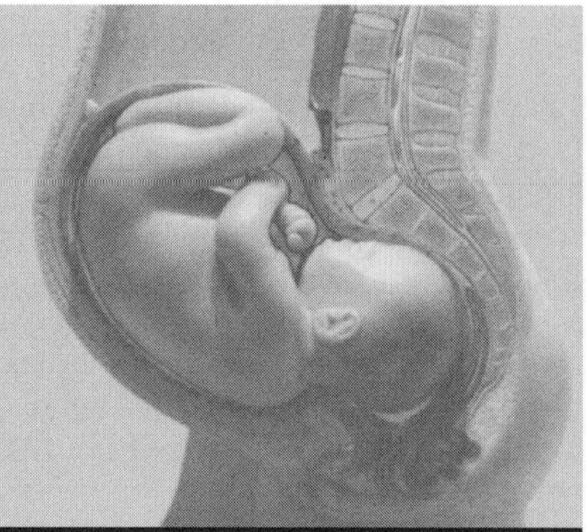

6 Puerperium

> **CASE 6A PUERPERAL SEPSIS**
>
> P_1L_0
> Delivered at home 4 days back
> FTVD conducted by dai. H/o leaking P/V 2 days
> Delivered dead baby. Delivery was difficult.
> Had PPH with retained placenta. Was taken to a nursing home where placenta was removed under GA
> Received 2 units blood
> Now c/o fever for 2 days high grade
> C/o vaginal foul smelling discharge
>
> *O/E:* Conscious, oriented
> Febrile: Temp 102°F
> Pallor ++
> No icterus
> Pulse: 120/min
> BP: 110/70 mmHg
> No Lymphadenopathy
> Breast: NAD (No mastitis)
> Chest/CVS: NAD
> Legs: No calf tenderness (No evidence of DVT)

Q1. What is puerperium?

Puerperium is the period of 6 weeks from the end of the third stage of labour (i.e. when the placenta is delivered) to the return of pre-pregnant state of normal health and activity.

Q2. The case sheet records that the uterine size is 20 weeks. Why is it important to record the uterine size after delivery?

After delivery the uterus undergoes involution, i.e. its size decreases almost to the pre-pregnancy size. Immediately after delivery, the fundus of the uterus is at the level of umbilicus (symphysio-fundal height 18–20 cm) and by 2 weeks, it decreases at the rate of 1–2 cm per day to become a pelvic organ (12 weeks size uterus, no longer palpable abdominally). By 6 weeks, its size decreases to the nonpregnant multiparous size, i.e. slightly larger than the nulliparous size.

When the rate of involution is slower than normal (clinically size of uterus is larger than expected during puerperium) it is known as *subinvolution* of the uterus, the commonest causes of the which are puerperal sepsis and/ or retained placental tissue. Retained placental fragments can be a cause of puerperal sepsis.

Q3. What should be the advise at time of discharge so that patient does not have infection?

The mother can usually be sent home by the next day. She should be encouraged to breast-feed and learn to care for her infant. Any discomfort due to breast engorgement is usually relieved by good bra support and analgesia. Analgesics may also be required to relieve the pain associated with the uterine contractions that continue after birth. Women who are unable to breastfeed or prefer to bottle feed should be given drugs to suppress lactation, otherwise breast abscess or mastitis can develop.

Patients who have undergone episiotomy should be instructed to clean the area at least twice a day with dilute antiseptic solution like Savlon or Dettol. Washing should be done from front to back, never the other way, to prevent infection. Additionally, local antiseptic creams such as Soframycin, Metrogyl gel or betadine should be applied twice daily to prevent infection and if necessary, oral antibiotics should be prescribed. For relieving pain, hot Sitz baths, hot water washes or hot water bag can be advised or analgesis tablets and/or xylocaine ointment can be prescribed.

Q4. Can a normal puerperium be associated with any problems?

Yes, the common puerperal problems are pain from episiotomy, difficulty in micturition, especially in first 24 hours, which may require catheterisation, constipation, mastitis (due to failure to express milk from one part of the breast) which may be complicated by staphylococcal infection, backache and psychological problems (the third day blues in which the mother becomes temporarily sad and emotional).

Serious puerperal problems include episiotomy wound disruption (gaped

P/A: Uterus 20 weeks
Soft
tender
No hepatosplenomegaly
No free fluid
No s/s of peritonitis

L/E: Old perineal tear at 6 o' clock, infected with purulent discharge

P/V: Vagina hot
Cervix patulous
Uterus 20 weeks, B/L fornices thick and tender
No fullness in POD (pouch of douglas)

Diagnosis:
P_1L_0 on 4th Postpartum day with puerperal pyrexia due to puerperal sepsis

Investigations
Complete Hemogram
LFT & KFT
Blood Culture
High vaginal and Endocervical swab for c/s
Midstream or catheter specimen of urine
USG examination to detect any retained placental tissue

Treatment
- Tab paracetamol 6 hourly
- Inj ampicillin 2 g IV every 6 hours, and
- Inj gentamicin 2 mg/kg body weight I/V followed by 1.5 mg/kg every 8 hours, and
- Inj metronidazole 500 mg IV every 8 hours
- Inj tetanus toxoid
- IV fluids
- Intake/output charting

episiotomy) which presents 2–3 weeks into the puerperium, puerperal pyrexia, puerperal sepsis, postpartum haemorrhage, postnatal anaemia, deep vein thrombosis (DVT), disseminated intravascular coagulation (DIC) and postnatal psychosis.

Q5. What should be done in a case of gaped episiotomy?

Depending on severity of infection, the wound may be managed from the OPD by prescribing oral antibiotics, sitz bath and local antiseptic creams like metrogyl, betadine, etc. After the wound becomes healthier, resuturing is done under local anesthesia after freshening the edges. Single layer closure is done by applying interrupted stitches using nonabsorbable or delayed-absorbable sutures.

Q6. What should be done in a case of deep vein thrombosis?

The patient should be readmitted to the hospital for intravenous heparin treatment. Heparin IV is started and the dose is adjusted to keep PTTK at around 2 times normal. Within 24 hours of the heparin, oral warfarin is started but the heparin infusion is not stopped till warfarin has been administered for 2–5 days. The dose of warfarin is adjusted so that the prothrombin time remains at 2–3 times the control. The heparin infusion is then stopped and the patient is discharged on oral warfarin which is continued for 3 months.

Q7. Would not warfarin result in uterine bleeding, since the uterus is still bulky?

No, because the patient usually reports after 2 weeks by the time when the uterus involutes and becomes a pelvic organ. The retracted uterus does not bleed and therefore warfarin does not cause uterine bleeding when administered as above.

Q8. Will any fever during puerperium be called puerperal pyrexia?

A patient is said to have puerperal pyrexia only if it occurs *after* the first 24 hours of puerperium and the oral temperature rises to 38°C or higher.

Q9. If the fever occurs within the first 24 hours of delivery, should we ignore it?

Normally yes, but not always. A low-grade temperature elevation is very common in the early postpartum period, particularly in the first 24 hours. Its causes include dehydration, tissue trauma and breast engorgement. However, it can be due to sepsis too, especially if the woman has had a premature rupture of membranes or a prolonged labour. In such cases, fever within the first 24 hours should not be taken lightly.

Q10. What is the difference between puerperal pyrexia and puerperal sepsis?

Puerperal sepsis is a septicemia that occurs after delivery due to bacterial infection spreading from the genital tract. Its symptoms and signs usually appear more than 24 hours after delivery. Puerperal sepsis occurs mostly due to the use of unclean hands or instruments but can also occur due to commensals that reach the genital tract from the bowel and urinary tract. Its incidence can be reduced by observing strict asepsis during delivery, minimizing the number of vaginal examinations and the trauma during labour, and by isolating infected patients.

Puerperal sepsis is one of the several causes of ***puerperal pyrexia,*** the others being UTI, mastitis, or less commonly, thrombophlebitis or respiratory tract infections.

Q11. How do we know whether or not the puerperal pyrexia is due to puerperal sepsis?

When fever during puerperium is associated with evidence of genital tract infection like offensive/purulent discharge, uterine tenderness, subinvolution of uterus, pelvic tenderness and infected wounds, then we know that it is due to puerperal sepsis. If s/s of other infections like UTI, chest infection, mastitis, etc. are present then these may be the cause of fever. Sometimes no specific s/s may be there then infections like typhoid, malaria, tuberculosis, etc. may be responsible and need to be ruled out.

Q12. What treatment/procedures other than mentioned in the case history may be required in a case of puerperal sepsis?

- Removal of all stitches if the wound is infected.
- Drainage of any abscess.

A laporotomy and possibly a hysterectomy is indicated, if peritonitis and subinvolution of the uterus are present, and there is no response to the measures detailed above. If there is no improvement with the above management and general peritonitis develops, a laparotomy will be performed to drain pus. If the uterus is necrotic and septic, a subtotal hysterectomy may be necessary.

Q13. The case sheet records that the patient does not have s/s of peritonitis. What are the signs and symptoms of peritonitis?

Peritonitis is diagnosed by the following symptoms and signs:

1. Fever/chills,
2. Nausea/vomiting,
3. Abdominal pain and rebound tenderness,
4. Distended abdomen,
5. Absent bowel sounds,
6. Shock.

Q14. The patient has foul smelling lochia. What is lochia? Is the lochia normally odorless? Is foul-smelling lochia a matter of concern?

Lochia is a vaginal discharge in the postnatal period. For first 4 days, lochia comprises mainly blood and remnants of trophoblastic tissue. Over the next week, its colour is reddish-brown and finally then changes to yellow. Occasionally, the lochia may become red again for a few days due to dissolution of clots leading to bleeding. A foul-smelling lochia could be due to retained placental tissue.

Q15. Why was this patient given tetanus toxoid injections?

The patient delivered at home and the details of her antenatal care was unknown. She was given an injection of tetanus toxoid as she might not have received it earlier.

Q16. How do you diagnose and manage retained placental tissue?

Retained placental tissue is suspected if the uterus is soft and bulky, and the lochia is excessive, foul-smelling and contain blood clots. The diagnosis is confirmed by USG examination. The placental tissue and clots are removed by digital exploration of the uterus. Ovum forceps or a large curette may also be used. Evacuation is done in labour room under sedation if required. However, if complete or the major bulk of the placenta is retained, the cervical os is closed, or the case follows a Cesarean section, then the procedure is done under general anesthesia.

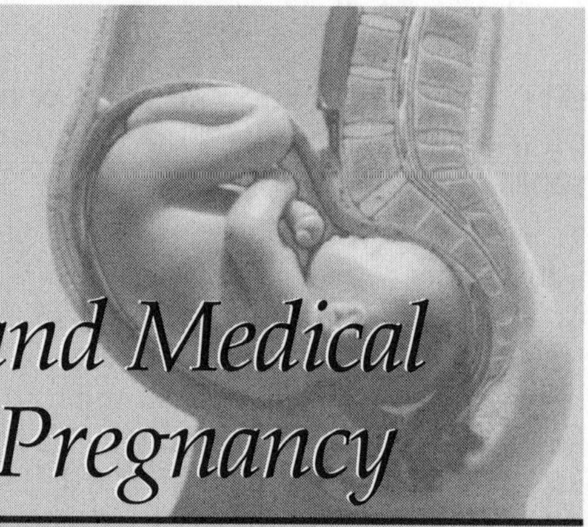

7 Contraception and Medical Termination of Pregnancy

CASE 7A CONTRACEPTIVE ADVICE

A 25-year-old P_1L_1
Had FTNVD 5 months back
Lactational
Having menstruation for last 2 months
Has come to Gynae OPD for contraception (wants to delay second pregnancy for 2–3 years)
Menstrual history: Normal cycles, no dysmenorrhoea or menorrhagia
LMP: 5 days back
Obstetrical history: FTNVD 6 months back. Pregnancy uneventful
Past History: No history of HT, diabetes, tuberculosis or anyother medical/surgical illness.
No h/o STDs or RTIs
Family history: No h/o HT, diabetes, malignancies.
Personal history: Educated (Graduate)

O/E: General examination: Normal
BP: 120/80 mmHg, Weight: 50 kg
P/A: NAD
P/S: Cervix, Vaginal healthy
P/V: Uterus R/V, small, soft, mobile, B/L fornices free.

Q1. What contraceptive advice will you give to this woman?

The history and examination suggest that she has no contraindications for any of the temporary contraceptive methods. Therefore she, along with her husband, should be informed about all the temporary contraceptive methods available (as mentioned below). This is known as *cafeteria approach.* They should be informed about hormonal contraceptives (oral and non-oral), IUDs, barrier methods and fertility awareness based methods (based on the knowledge of ovulation and thus period of fertility around it). Thereafter, we discuss with the couple and help them to choose a method is most suited to them. We recommend to them the hormonal method and IUDs as these have lower failure rate and inform them of their advantages and disadvantages. Once the couple decides on a method, we inform them in detail about it.

Q2. Would you recommend lactational amenorrhea method to anyone?

Yes, but only when all the following conditions are satisfied viz.,

1. The woman is amenorrheic and <6 months postpartum;

2. The infant is on exclusive breastfeeding or gets at least 85% of feeds as breastmilk;
3. The mother breastfeeds her child at least 8–10 times in a day and at least once at night, and
4. No daytime feeding is regularly >4 hours apart and no night feeding is >6 hours apart.

Q3. When can a normal menstruating woman get an IUD inserted?

She can have a copper-bearing IUD inserted at any time within the first 12 days after the start of menstrual bleeding or at any other time if it is certain that she is not pregnant. IUDs are contraindicated in cervical/ endometrial cancer or unexplained vaginal bleeding, in recent pelvic infection, and in uterine distortions that impede correct IUD placement. There should be a follow-up check-up 3–6 weeks following insertion.

Q4. Should an IUD be inserted immediately after delivery or abortion?

Yes, but it should not be done in cases of sepsis. If it is not inserted immediately after abortion, then it should be inserted after 4 weeks of abortion.

After delivery, it can be placed immediately (within 48 hrs) but the technique of insertion is different from the usual one and expulsion rate is more. It is preferable to insert it 4 weeks after delivery.

Q5. What will you do if a woman using a copper-bearing IUD is found to be pregnant?

If a woman conceive with IUCD, we first exclude ectopic pregnancy. If it is an intrauterine pregnancy and the CuT thread is visible, the CuT should be removed. Continuing pregnancy with CuT *in situ* carries the risk of septic abortion and preterm delivery. If the IUD thread is not visible, we do an USG to locate the CuT: If it is not visible then we assume it was expelled. If it is visible in the uterus then we explain to the patient the risk and advise her an MTP. If she decides to continue the pregnancy, we ask her to report immediately if she has heavy bleeding, cramping, pain, abnormal vaginal discharge, or fever.

Q6. Which is the commonest used OP for contraception?

This is low dose combined oral contraceptive (COC) pill. Mala D/Mala N are supplied in a pack of 28 tablets containing 21 hormonal tablets and 7 non-hormonal tablets containing Ferrous Fumerate. Hormonal tablets contain 30 µg of Ethinyl estradiol and 0.15 mg of Levonorgestrel. Mala N is supplied free of charge by Government under Family Planning Program while Mala D is made available by the Govt at subsidized rates. Newer pack is started immediately after first pack is over.

Q7. Are contraceptive pills safe for women?

Not always. Because of estrogen content they are contraindicated in liver diseases, breast cancer, migraine and thromboembolic disease. They should also not be used if there is a possibility that the woman is pregnant. Hence, women using pills should be called after the 3 months for a check-up, and thereafter, for an annual check-up. Women on POPs or implants do not require annual checkups.

Contraceptive pills also have a few beneficial effects: They regularize the cycle, limits blood loss, and alleviates dysmenorrhea and premenstrual tension. They lower the risk of endometrial and ovarian cancer and benign diseases of the breast and ovary. The also prevent pelvic inflammatory disease and improve bone mineral density.

Q8. Can a woman start combined oral contraceptives (COCs) at any time?

Yes, provided she is sure that she is not pregnant. In such cases additional contraceptive protection is required for the next 7 days. It is best to start COCs within 5 days after the start of her menstrual bleeding. Since pills decrease the milk production, postpartum women should not use COCs for the first 6 months. If she is not breastfeeding, COCs can be started 21 days or more after delivery. Breastfeeding women can take minipill (progestogen only pill).

Q9. What should a woman do if she misses one dose of combined oral contraceptives (COCs)?

If the woman misses 1 or 2 pills (hormonal), she should take one pill as soon as she remembers it. She should also take the pill scheduled for the day and continue with the subsequent routine of daily pills. If the woman misses 3 or more pills, she should take one pill immediately and then continue with one pill daily. Till 7 pills have been taken continuously, she should take additional precaution like barrier contraception or abstinence. Emergency contraception may be taken if 3 or more pills missed in the first row. If 3 or more pills missed in 3rd row, take all the pills in the row as above but discard the last row (placebo or iron tablets) and start the new pack next day. If the iron pills (4th row) are missed, she should discard the missed pills and continue the rest.

Q10. What are the other combined contraceptive pills available?

1. *Very low dose pills:* Contain Ethinyl estradiol 20 µg with Desogestrel 15 mg
2. *Triphasic pills:* Contain 21 pills in which doses of estrogen and progestin vary according to the cycle so that minimum doses are given.
3. *Pills with newer progestins:* These pills contain newer progestin Drospirenone 3 mg along with estrogen. It is a spironolactone derivative and has antiandrogenic and antimineralocorticoid properties. Use of DSP containing OCP is associated with less water retention and thus less weight gain than traditional COCs. This also improves acne, hirsutism and PMS.

Q11. Saheli is a much-advertized contraceptive. What does it contain and how does it act?

Saheli contains *centchroman* (30 mg/tablet) which is a nonsteroidal oral contraceptive. It exhibits a potent antiestrogenic activity. It is started in a dose of 30 mg (1 tablet) on the first day of menstruation, given twice a week for the first 3 months and then once weekly. It is safe and reliable and its failure rate (1.6 HWY) is comparable to that of OC pills. It inhibits implantation of blastocyst, alters tubal motility and reduces the sperm penetration of cervical mucous. Being nonsteroidal, it has none of the major side effects of steroidal contraceptives. Menstrual disturbances like oligomenorrhea and amenorrhea are found in more than a third of the users.

Q12. What are the indications of progesterone-only methods of hormonal contraception?

These are recommended to women in whom oestrogens are contraindicated or not tolerated. They suppress ovulation, thicken the cervical mucus, and cause involution of endometrium making it hostile for implantation. There are oral, subcutaneous, intramuscular, intrauterine and intravaginal routes of administration for progestogen only contraceptives.

Q13. What is the contraceptive pill which contains only progestogen? Is it prescribed in the same way as Mala D?

This is progestogen only pill (POP) also known as Minipill, containing Desogestrel 75 µg. It is supplied in a pack of 28 tablets. The pill should be started within first 5 days of start of menstruation, taken everyday at the same time without any break. If started after first 5 days, then additional contraception should be used for two days. If woman is more than 12 hrs late in taking pill, she should take pill immediately and use backup for 2 days.

After delivery, minipills can be started at any time if non-breastfeeding. In breast-feeding females, progestogen only pills can be started after 6 weeks. Breakthrough bleeding occurs in 20–30 percent cases. Failure rate is high but for breast-feeding women and premenopausal women they are very effective.

Q14. If couple asks for contraception after an unprotected act of sexual intercourse, can we help them?

Yes, in such a situation and also in cases of method failure like condom rupture or forgotten contraceptive pills, we can give Emergency Contraceptive pill also known as Morning After Pill. This is available in the form of Single pill(I-Pill) containing 1.5 mg of levonorgestrel or A pack of Two Pills (E-Pill) containing 0.75 mg LNG in each tablets. Pill is to be taken within 5 days, preferably within 72 hrs after unprotected intercourse.

Q15. If emergency contraceptive pill is not available, can the standard oral contraceptive pills be used for the same purspose?

Yes, she can take combined estrogen-progestogen pills in 2 doses (low dose COC Pills: 2 doses of 4 tablets each 12 hours apart). Main side effect with this regimen is vomitings.

Q16. Can any other method be used for emergency contraception apart from pills.

Yes. Cu-IUD can be inserted within 5 days of unprotected intercourse if no contra-indications for IUD are there and woman desires continuing contraception with IUD.

Q17. What are different methods of female sterilisation procedures?

1. *Laparoscopic tubal ligation* using Falope's rings. This is the most commonly used method for female sterilization.
2. *Minilaparotomy:* A midline vertical or transverse suprapubic 3–4 cm incision is given. This is done when incision is required only for the surgical procedure of tubal ligation.
3. *Laparotomy:* When abdomen is already opened for any other procedure like cesarean section, ovarian cyst, rupture uterus, etc. tubal ligation can be done concurrently.

Tubal ligation can be done at any of the following times:

i. *Interval procedure:* In a normal menstruating woman during first 10 days or at any other time when it is certain that she is not pregnant. Laparoscopic ligation is preferable over open procedure but if instruments are not available or any contraindications for laparoscopic procedure are there, then open minilap ligation can be done.
ii. *Postabortion:* Can be done with first and second trimester MTPs. Laparoscopic ligation is preferable concurrent with first trimester MTP while in second trimester MTP minilap ligation is preferred.
iii. *Postpartum:* Immediately after delivery,
iv. In cases of cesarean section, tubal ligation is done in the same sitting after closing the uterine incision.

Q18. What is Postpartum Sterilization?

Postpartum sterilization (PPS), is minilap ligation procedure done after delivery when woman is still in the hospital. PPS can be done as soon as patient has recovered from the stress and exhaustion of labour. Usually done next day after delivery. Can be done up to 7 days postpartum preferably within 72 hr after delivery. During this time, the uterus is palpable in the abdomen and tubes are easily approachable through a small incision. PPS can be performed under general, regional or local anesthesia.

PPS is contraindicated in severe pre-eclampsia/eclampsia, puerperal fever, severe antepartum or postpartum haemorrhage, and severe trauma to the genital tract at time of delivery. If PPS is not done within 7 days of delivery, then if required, ligation should be done after 6 weeks.

Q19. Can there be sterilization failure in females?

Yes, the common causes of female sterilization failure are:

1. An undetected luteal phase pregnancy that was present at the time of sterilization;
2. Mistaken occlusion of a structure other than the fallopian tube (most often, the round ligament);
3. Incomplete or inadequate occlusion of the fallopian tubes;
4. Misplacement of the mechanical device; and
5. Development of tuboperitoneal fistula.

Q20. Should sterilization be done on anyone who requests it?

No, the Govt of India has stipulated certain eligibility criteria for sterilization:

1. The client must be married;
2. Male clients should preferably be below the age of 60 years;
3. Female client should be below the age of 45 years and above 22 years;
4. The couple should have at least one child whose age is above one year.
5. Clients or their spouses must not have undergone sterilization in the past, unless it is a case of sterilization failure.
6. Clients must be in a perfectly normal state of mind so as to understand the full implication of sterilization;
7. Mentally ill clients must be certified by a psychiatrist, and consent in such cases should be given by legal guardian/spouse;
8. The client must be informed of all the available methods of family planning and must make an informed decision for sterilization voluntarily.

Q21. Is the consent of spouse required for sterilization procedures?

No such consent is required.

Q1. How do you define medical termination of pregnancy?

Medical termination of pregnancy (MTP) is induced abortion under the MTP Act, whether it is done surgically or medically.

Q2. What is the MTP Act?

India was the first country to have a family planning program and the MTP Act of India was enacted in 1971 to check the rising incidences of criminal abortions. The act defines when the MTP can be done, the person who should do it, the place where it should be done, and the indications for which it should be done. As per the act:

1. An MTP can be done anytime from the day of conception till 20 weeks of gestation.
2. The MTP should be done by a person with 6 months of house job or diploma or MD degree course in obstetrics and gynecology or if he has assisted a RMP in the performance of twenty five cases of MTP in a hospital established or maintained or a training institution approved for this purpose, by the Government.
3. The MTP should be done at a place that is registered under the act, i.e a government institution or a place approved by director of health services.
4. The indications of MTP include:
   a. In order to save the life of the pregnant woman.
   b. In order to prevent grave injury to the physical or mental health of the pregnant woman.
   c. In view of the substantial risk that the child if born would suffer from such physical or mental abnormalities to be seriously handicapped.
   d. As the pregnancy is alleged by pregnant woman to have been caused by rape.
   e. As the pregnancy has occurred as a result of failure of a contraceptive device or methods used by the couple.

CASE 7B FIRST TRIMESTER MTP

30 years Mrs X
$P_{2+0+0+2}$ Last child birth: 1 year back, Not lactating

C/o amenorrhoea 2 months, associated with nausea
Wants termination of pregnancy
H/o urine pregnancy test positive 1 week back.
Menstrual history: Cycles: 3/30 days regular, LMP: 2 month back

Obstetrical history: P_2L_2

Ist: FTNVD 3 years back, baby alive, healthy and immunized
2nd: FTNVD 1 year back, baby alive, healthy and immunized
Not desirous of further pregnancy

Contraceptive history:
Couple using barrier contraceptive

O/E:
GC fair
Pallor: nil
P: 80/min, BP: 110/74 mmHg
Chest & CVS: NAD

P/A: Soft, NAD

P/S: Cx bluish, vagina congested, No discharge

P/V: Cx ↓, soft, uterus AV, soft, 8 weeks size, mobile, non-tender, fornices free

Diagnosis: G_3 $P_{2+0+0+2}$ with 8 weeks pregnancy for MTP

Indication for MTP: Contraceptive failure (barrier contraceptive)

Adv:
Hb
Urine alb, sugar

Counselling for contraception giving different choices

Plan: MTP with ligation/IUCD insertion (if either of these chosen by the couple) under IV sedation and local anaesthesia after taking proper consent.

Q3. When would you refuse to do a medical termination of pregnancy? Does not contraceptive failure offer a convenient excuse for MTP anytime?

Whenever termination of pregnancy is not in accordance with the above mentioned criteria, MTP will not be performed. Also, MTP will be refused *if it does not have the consent* of the pregnant woman.

Contraceptive failure is often not a 'convenient excuse'. If pregnancy results from contraceptive failure, the anguish caused by such unwanted pregnancy sometimes constitutes a grave injury to the mental health of the pregnant woman and is a valid justification for termination of pregnancy. We will also not terminate any pregnancy if it is likely to be for female foeticide after prenatal sex determination. Hence one has to be very careful in determining the exact indication in second trimester pregnancy terminations.

Q4. Are there any precautions to be taken for doing MTP?

When the patient comes to us, we take history, do a general and gynecological examination to confirm the pregnancy and ascertain the period of gestation. We estimate the haemoglobin and urine albumin/sugar in all pateints. For primigravida, we also test the blood group. Ultrasound is performed if necessary. If there are no contraindications to MTP (Hb < 8 g%, suspected ectopic pregnancy, undiagnosed adenexal mass, uncontrolled BP >160/100 mmHg), the client is given MTP No. to maintain the confidentiality after filling forms I and C. The choice of the MTP method depends on the period of gestation and the client's will.

Q5. How is MTP done in the first trimester?

The MTP can be done either medically or surgically.

Medical abortion is noninvasive method for MTP till 7 weeks of gestation and does not result in anaesthetic and operative complications. However, it is not indicated in anemic patients (Hb <8 g%) as it takes longer and the patient may bleed for more than 7 days. It is also contraindicated if there is serious medical illness like renal and liver disease, allergy to drugs, and if the patient in noncompliant

Surgical evacuation is done till 12 weeks, either by suction evacuation (electrical), or manual vacuum aspiration (MVA). WHO recommends MVA (manual vacuum aspiration) instead of suction evacuation. The complications of the surgical evacuation include:

1. Anesthetic complications,
2. Excessive bleeding,
3. Tear of the cervix,
4. Perforation of the uterus.
5. Perforation of the bowel: The uterus is so soft that the cannula goes through-and-through the uterus and sucks the bowel too.

Incidence of perforation of uterus during suction evacuation is 5%.

Q6. How is a 'medical' abortion done in the first trimester?

In april 2002, the drug controller of India approved mifepristone and misoprostol for MTP of 7 weeks or less gestation.

After counseling the client, we give mifepristone (RU486 - an antiprogesterone drug) 200 mg orally on day 1. This results in embryo death. 48 hours after administration of mifepristone (day 3), we give 400 microgram Misoprost (PG-E1 analogue) orally or intravaginally. We observe the patient for 6 hours, by the end of which the patient usually aborts. Before she leaves the clinic, a P/V is done: If os is open or products of conception are felt in the cervical canal, digital evacuation is done. The patient is sent home and counseled that she might bleed longer in medical MTP. She can do routine work. On day 15, ultrasound is done again to look for any residual conceptus. If present, she needs surgical evacuation to remove those products.

Q7. How is a 'surgical' abortion done in the first trimester?

Surgical abortion is commonly and preferably used for 1st trimester MTP. It is usually done by suction and evacuation (S and E). It can also be done by dilatation and curettage (D and C) though this is not widely used nowadays.

It is important here to understand the difference between S and E and D and C. The term **suction and evacuation** actually refers to the *dilatation* of the cervix, *evacuation* of the conceptus by suction and finally a *check curettage* to check for the completeness of evacuation. The term **dilatation and curettage**, when used in the context of MTP, refers to the *dilatation* of the cervix followed by *evacuation* of the conceptus by ovum forceps, and finally *check curettage* to check for completeness of evacuation. Hence, the essential difference between S and E and D and C, in the context of MTP, is whether the evacuation is done by by suction or by instruments. Suction is easier, more reliable, and is associated with less bleeding.

Q8. If curettage is always done at the end to check for the completeness of the evacuation, why cannot it be used for removing of the conceptus too?

Compared to the curette, the suction canula or the products of conception forceps are better instruments for removing the products of conception from the uterine cavity. It is quite difficult to remove the conceptus completely by curettage. The curettage only tells us whether the conceptus has been removed completely: It gives a gritty feeling against the uterine wall when the evacuation is complete.

Q9. How is a suction evacuation (S and E) done?

Suction evacuation is done either by using an electrical suction machine or by manual vacuum aspiration (MVA), i.e. by applying suction using the vacuum syringe. The procedure is done in minor OT under local or regional anesthesia, and under full asepsis.

After dilatation of cervix with Hegar's dilator, a plastic canula (the Karman's canula) is introduced and suction is applied to it. By too and fro movements of cannula, evacuation is completed followed by a *check curettage* and IV methergine 0.25 mg. The evacuation is assumed to be complete when no products but only bubbles are obtained on suction, and when there is a feel of the contracted uterine cavity over the canula and the uterine walls present a gritty surface.

Canulas of different sizes are used for terminating pregnancies of different durations. For convenience, the canulas are numbered 4 to 12 to indicate the duration of pregancy (in weeks) for which their use is recommended. Thus, for an MTP in the 8th week, the No.8 canula is used.

MVA creates the same amount of suction pressure as that of electrical suction machine. Yet, it is safer than electrical suction machine because it has a mechanism of releasing the vacuum as soon as perforation of uterus occurs so that bowel injuries are less as compared to suction evacuation. It is safe even in the hands of paramedicals. It also has the advantage that there is no need for electricity and it is very useful at peripheral health centers.

Q10. Do you prefer local or regional anesthesia for surgical evacuation?

Local anesthesia is preferred for the surgical evacuations. Sometimes when cervical os is tightly closed and dilatation is going to be difficult, regional or general anesthesia may be required as in nulliparous woman or with previous cesarean section. But nowadays with the option of cervical dilatation with misoprostol tablet given 2–4 hours before procedure, the requirement of anaesthesia is even less.

Q11. What is menstrual regulation? Why is it not considered as an abortion?

Menstrual regulation is early abortion within 44 days of amenorrhea with a syringe. It was widely used when sensitive tests for diagnosing pregnancy were not available and an MR used to be done on missing a period. Now we have very sensitive pregnancy diagnostic tests (requiring only a urine sample) so that very early pregnancy is diagnosed and accordingly patient is offered termination by various methods.

Menstrual regulation is not termed abortion as this OPD procedure is performed whenever periods are delayed up to 44 days without confirming pregnancy. As mentioned above, this used to be performed earlier but not done nowadays as sensitive pregnancy tests are available. The problem with MR is that lot of procedures used to be performed in nonpregnant cases unnecessarily.

Q12. How is 'medical' abortion done in the second trimester?

There are several methods for *second trimester abortion*:

- Mifepristone (200 to 600 mg) is administered orally and wait for 48 hours after administering it. It causes intrauterine death (IUD) of the fetus. The uterus is then stimulated with Misoprost, 200 μg orally every 3 to 4 hours until the fetus is expelled or for maximum of 6 doses. It can also be administered by sublingual or intravaginal route.
- *Extra-aminiotic instillation of Ethacrydine lactate:* A Foley's catheter is inserted into the uterus beyond internal os and ethacrydine lactate (Emcredil), an antiseptic solution is instilled at a dose of 10 ml per week, i.e. we give 140 ml if it is a 14 weeks gestation. We then clamp the catheter and leave it in. The catheter is expelled when the cervix dilates: If it does not, then it is removed after 6 hours. Usually the patient gets spontaneous contractions and expels the fetus. If she does not, we try *augmentation* with escalating doses of IV oxytocin.
- We can also use prostaglandins which have the advantage that they are oxytocics and cause cervical ripening too. We can give PGF_2 alpha, PGE_2 *or* PGE_1.

For ripening only, cerviprime gel, i.e. PG-E_2 is used for intracervical instillation. If we put the gel for 6 hours, the cervix gets ripe and further it can supplemented by oxytocics for stimulating uterine contractions, or we can use PG-F_2 alpha 250 microgram intramuscularly every 3 to 4 hours for maximum of 10 doses. We can also put 2.5 mg of PG F_2 alpha intra-amniotically. Midtrimester abortion is less safe though safe methods are now available within the Act.

Q13. How is 'surgical' abortion done in the second trimester?

There are two 'surgical' methods of mid-trimester abortion. Suction evacuation preceded by cervical preparation can be performed only by an experienced performer and has very high complication risk. It is not preferred as safer medical methods are available. Abdominal hysterotomy is performed in patients who do not respond to medical methods or have contraindication to it.

Q14. Why is suction evacuation in second trimester associated with high risk?

By the second trimester, bony tissues are formed in the fetus and therefore it bleeds a lot and there are considerable chances of incomplete abortion if attempt is made to abort by suction evacuation. For proper evacuation cervix needs to be prepared (slow dilatation using mechanical dilators) followed by evacuation by experienced surgeon using special instruments for evacuation of the fetal parts. As this carries high risk or injuries, hemorrhage and incomplete evacuation, medical methods are preferred. In mid trimester medical abortion we have to ripen the cervix[1] and stimulate the uterus, as abortion at this gestation is like a minilabour.

Q15. What are the complications of mid-trimester medical abortion?

There can be rupture uterus due to prostaglandin-induced contractions. If rupture occurs, we have to open up the patient, take out the products of conception, repair the uterus and if required, perform hysterectomy. Other complications are haemorrhage, infection and incomplete abortion. Surgical evacuation can cause cervical trauma, uterine perforation and injury to intra-abdominal organs.

Q16. What is Feticide?

Feticide literally means killing of the fetus. More commonly, the term feticide refers to the termination of pregnancy when it is not allowable under the MTP Act. For example, if pregnancy is terminated after sex determination because couple does not want female child, it is female feticide. Also, termination beyond legal limits, i.e. 20 weeks, will be feticide if done for indications other than fetal defects not compatible with *ex utero* survival, e.g. anencephaly.

Cases with contraceptive failure would report in first trimester after missing one or two periods and are unlikely to report in 2nd trimester. However, there is no hard and fast rule that contraceptive failures cannot come in second trimester. Individual judgement and considerations are required in different cases. For example, second trimester MTPs are justified in cases of conception in lactational amenorrhoea or pregnancies in unmarried young girls. These are feticides, but as these are under valid indications, MTP term is used.

---

[1]Cervical ripening is a biochemical change. The cervix is normally tough and has a lot of collagen fibers. The cervix becomes soft. Dilatation and effacement of the cervix before labour is cervical ripening.

- Vaginal Discharge
- Menstrual Disorders and Menopause
- Infertility
- Uterovaginal Prolapse
- Urinary Symptoms
- Lump Abdomen
- Acute Pain Abdomen
- Gynaecological Oncology

Section 2

Gynaecology

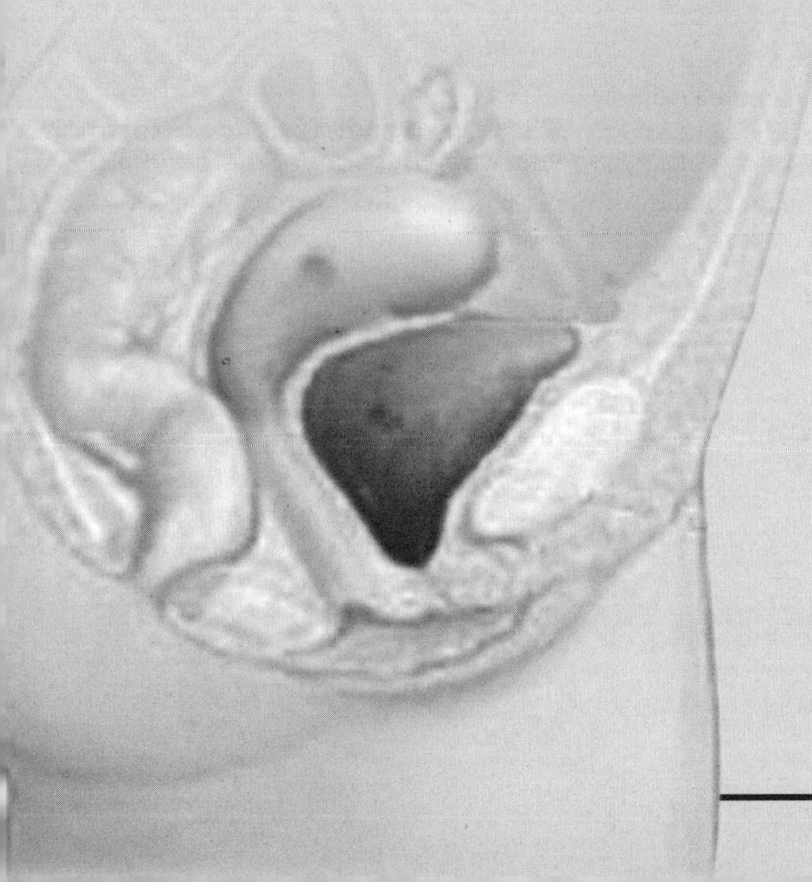

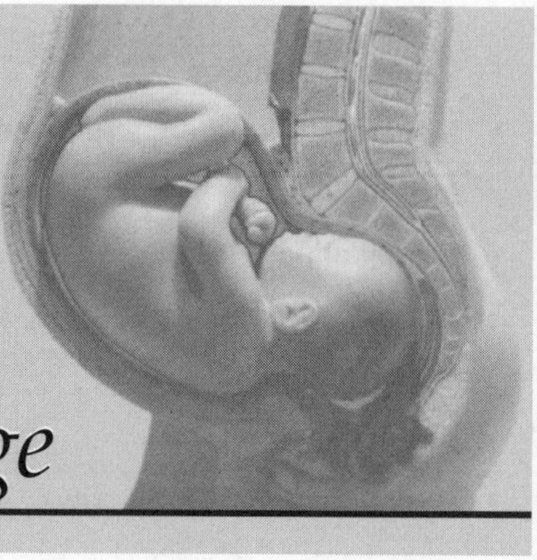

8 Vaginal Discharge

CASE 8A VAGINAL DISCHARGE (TRICHOMONAS VAGINITIS)

A 25-year-old Nulliparous woman, married for 1 month

C/o
Vaginal discharge for 10 days
Associated with itching vulva
Symptoms started after last menstrual period
LMP: 10 days back
No menstrual complaints, urinary complaints
No urogenital symptoms in the husband

O/E:
GC fair, afebrile
P/A: NAD

L/E: Itch marks present over vulva
Thin greenish discharge seen coming thro' introitus

P/S: Frothy thin greenish discharge
Strawberry patches seen on vagina and ectocervix
No discharge seen from cervical os

Q1. The patient has itching in the vulva. Are all types of vaginal discharge associated with itching?

No, *N.gonorrhoeae* or bacterial vaginosis do not result in itching until and unless there is mixed infection with *T.vaginalis* or *Candida*. If the vaginal discharge is itchy, it could be either *Trichomonas vaginalis or Monilial vaginitis*.

Q2. Can vaginal discharge be normal? If yes, when is it considered abnormal?

A small amount of vaginal discharge occurs normally due to hormonal changes. It is clear and odourless. The normal discharge varies during menstrual cycle and is more during ovulation. Normal discharge may increase if cervical erosion is present.

The term 'cervical erosion' is a misnomer: It is cervical ectopy, i.e. endocervical epithelium is present at ectopic site (ectocervix), i.e. the squamo-columnar junction descends onto ectocervix. It occurs under the influence of reproductive hormones, during pregnancy or after delivery.

The vaginal discharge is considered abnormal when its quantity, colour or odour is not normal.

Q3. Is it possible, by examination, to differentiate discharges of cervical and vaginal origin?

Yes, on per speculum examination vaginal discharge is seen smearing the vaginal walls. Cervical discharge is seen as mucopurulent or purulent discharge exuding from the cervical os.

Q4. How do we treat vaginal discharge if laboratory facilities are not available?

In such circumstances, we adopt the *syndromic approach*, a concept developed by WHO to treat the syndrome without waiting for lab tests reports. Syndromic management is treatment assuming that the infecting organism is the one most commonly responsible for each syndrome. Even when laboratory facilities are available, the tests require resources, add to the cost of treatment, may require clients to make extra visits to the clinic and almost always result in delays in treatment. For these reasons, syndromic management is widely used for syndromes such as vaginal discharge, lower abdominal pain, urethral discharge and genital ulcer even in developed countries with advanced laboratory facilities. WHO has developed simple algorithms to guide health care providers in using the syndromic approach. It is polytherapy but its advantage is that there are no dropouts for treatments, especially in treating STDs and can be administered even by paramedicals.

Q5. You recommend the syndromic approach when laboratory facilities are not available. What is syndromic approach for vaginal discharge?

Syndromic approach for vaginal discharge is that all women presenting with abnormal vaginal discharge should receive treatment for bacterial vaginosis and trichomoniasis. Additional treatment for candidal infection is

P/V: Cx ↓, uterus AV, NS, mobile, fornices free non tender.

Wet smear examination of vaginal discharge: Motile organisms (*Trichomonas vaginalis*) seen

Δ *Trichomonal vaginitis*

R_x

Metronidazole 400 mg bd for 7 days for both partners

indicated when clinically apparent (white, curd-like discharge, redness of the vulva and vagina, and itching).

Treatment for cervical infection should be added to the treatment for vaginitis if suspected (for example, if the patient's partner has a urethral discharge or high risk factors), or if signs of cervical infection (mucopurulent cervical discharge or easy bleeding) are seen on speculum examination. An important consideration in the syndromic approach for vaginal discharge is whether or not a speculum is available. The WHO algorithm for syndromic management of vaginal discharge is given in Flow Chart 8.1.

Q6. In case 8A, you have prescribed metronidazole to both partners. Do we always need to treat sexual partners in cases of vaginal infections?

No, not all infective agents causing vaginitis/ cervicitis are sexually transmitted. For candidal infection and bacterial vaginosis it is still debatable whether these are STIs or not, therefore the treatment of the partner is not required in these cases. Trichomoniasis, gonorrhoea and chlamydia are STDs and therefore the sexual partners should be treated in these cases.

Table 8.1

Type and cause	*Nature of discharge*	*Perspeculum examination*	*Laboratory test*	*Treatment*
Trichomonas vaginitis *Trichomonas vaginalis*, a protozoan. Commonly occurs in postmenstrual period when the resistance of vaginal epithelium is lowered due to alkaline pH of vagina.	Frothy, greenish, copious discharge which may be associated with vulval itching and soreness, dysuria, dyspareunia.	Frothy, thin discharge. Ectocervix and vagina show strawberry patches called strawberry cervicitis. Under colposcope, the strawberry patches appear as small punctations arranged in groups. Each punctation under high power (of colposcopy) has typical forked or Y-shaped vessels.	Wet smear under light microscope shows the *Trichomonas vaginalis* which looks bigger than WBC and is mobile by ameboid movements of its body. Though it has flagella but it does not move by its flagella; moreover in wet smear flagella cannot be appreciated. Vaginal pH-alkaline (>7).	First choice: Metronidazole 2 gm single oral dose or 400 mg BD × 7 days Alternative regimen Stat dose of Secnidazole or tinidazole (2 gm) or Tinidazole 500 mg bd × 5 days for both partners.
Monilial vaginitis *Candida albicans*, an opportunistic parasite.	Curdy white or cheesy and itchy.	Curdy white or cheesy discharge and inflamed vagina and cervix.	Smear with 10% KOH on a slide shows hyphae of the fungus under light microscope and is diagnostic of candidal vaginitis. Vaginal pH-acidic (<7).	First choice: Miconazole or Clotrimazole 200 mg vaginal pessary every day for 3 days or Clotrimazole 500 mg pessary single dose or Tab fluconazole 150 mg (oral) single dose Alternative regimen: **nystatin** 100 000 unit vaginal tablet, one a day for 14 days
Bacterial vaginosis Anaerobic organisms (*Gardenella vaginalis*, *Mycoplasma hominis*, mobilincus sp.)	Greyish-white discharge with a fishy-odor. Discharge sticks to the vaginal walls	Thin, white homogenous discharge coating the walls of the vagina. Characteristic discharge is copious and has a fishy odor	Vaginal pH becomes less acidic (7.0) because of replacement of lacto-bacillli in vagina. Wet smear shows epithelial cells with their borders obscured by several adherent bacteria. These cells are called clue cells	First choice: Metron dazole 2 gm single oral dose or 400 mg BD × 7 days. Alternative regimen clindamycin 300 mg bid for 7 days

Contd....

Contd....

Chlamydia trachomatis Cervicitis	Mucopurulent discharge Asymptomatic in 80% cases		Detected by PCR, NAAT (nucleic acid amplification technique) from the secretions. EIAs and direct fluoroscent antibody testing can also be used as diagnostic tests. These tests are expensive and are not available routinely.	First choice azithromycin 1 g orally in a single dose or Doxycycline 100 mg BD × 7 days. Alternative regimen Ofloxacin 400 mg bd × 7 days or Tetracycline/erythromycin 500 mg QID × 7 days
Gonococcal cervicitis Gram –ve dipplococci. *N.gonorrhoeae*	Purulent vaginal discharge. Asymptomatic in 50% cases	Cervix looks angry, red and exudes pus along with urethritis.	Pus Gram staining confirms the diagnosis.	First choice cefixime 400 mg oral single dose or Cefitriaxone (MONOCEF) 250 mg IM stat. Alternative regimen Ciprofloxacillin 500 mg orally as single dose. Or spectinomycin 2 gm IM single inj.

Doxycycline, tetracycline, ciprofloxacin, ofloxacin and fluconazole should be avoided in pregnancy and when breastfeeding.

For bacterial vaginosis anc trichomoniasis treatment should be *Preferably delayed after first trimester.* **Metronidazolea** 200 or 250 mg orally 3 times a day for 7 days, or **metronidazole** gel 0.75%, one full applicator (5 g) intravaginally twice a day for 5 days, or **clindamycin** 300 mg orally twice a day for 7 days

Flow Chart 8.1

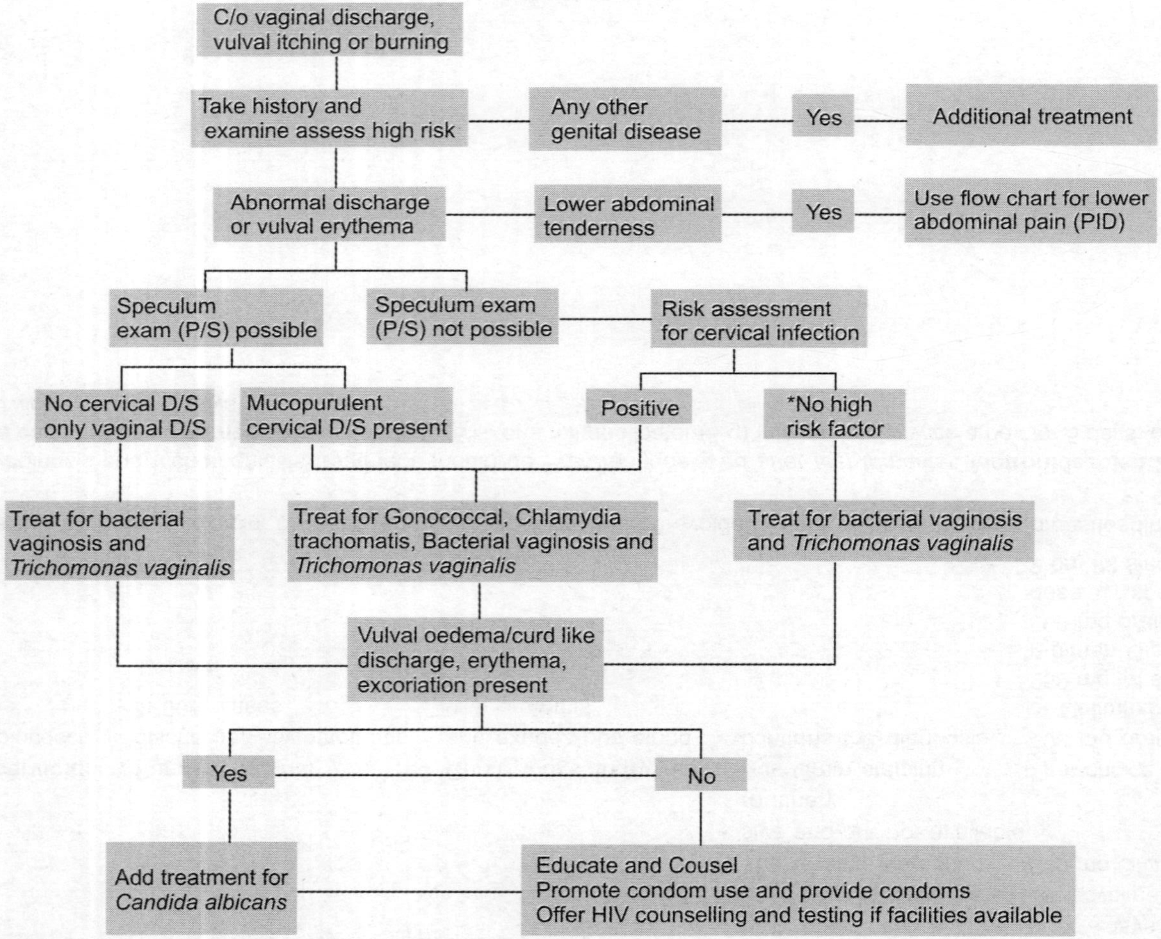

* Risk assessment for cervical infection requiring treatment is positive if:

1. History
   - Her partner has symptoms
   - She is a sex worker
   - She thinks she was exposed to an STI
2. If she comes from an area that is known to have a high prevalence of gonorrhoea and chlamydia
3. If speculum exam reveals:
   - Mucopurulent discharge
   - Cervix bleeds easily when touched

Q7. If lab facilities are available, how do you collect vaginal discharge for testing and what tests can be done on vaginal discharge?

For vaginal discharge take a sample of discharge from the side walls or deep in the vagina where discharge pools (or use discharge remaining on speculum). Diagnosing vaginal infections is very easy and can be done with simple tests with minimum lab facilities.

pH testing: Touch pH paper to discharge on swab or speculum and note pH.

Microscopic examination of the wet mount sample: This is a very simple OPD procedure, can aid in diagnosis of yeast infection (*Candida albicans*), Bacterial vaginosis and trichomoniasis. For this mix specimen of discharge with 1 or 2 drops of saline on a glass slide and cover with a coverslip. Examine at 100X magnification and look for typical jerky movement of motile trichomonads. Examine at 40X magnification to look for yeast cells. To make identification of yeast cells easier in wet mount slides, mix the vaginal swab in another drop of saline and add a drop of 10% potassium hydroxide to dissolve other cells. Clue cells are seen in bacterial vaginosis.

Gram stain microscopy: A Gram stain slide can be prepared at the same time as the wet. mount by rolling the swab on a separate slide and subsequently doing Gram staining.

Q8. Are there any complications of untreated vaginal discharge?

Yes, but not in all types of vaginal discharge. *Bacterial vaginosis* is associated with complications during pregnancy (premature rupture of membranes, preterm labour, chorioamnionitis, puerperial sepsis) and non-pregnant state (PID, post hysterectomy vaginal cuff cellulitis). *Chlamydial infection* can cause PID and later on tubal blockage and infertility, and perihepatitis (Fitz-Hugh-Curtis- syndrome). *Gonococcal cervicitis* result in acute pelvic inflammatory disease in 25% of the cases.

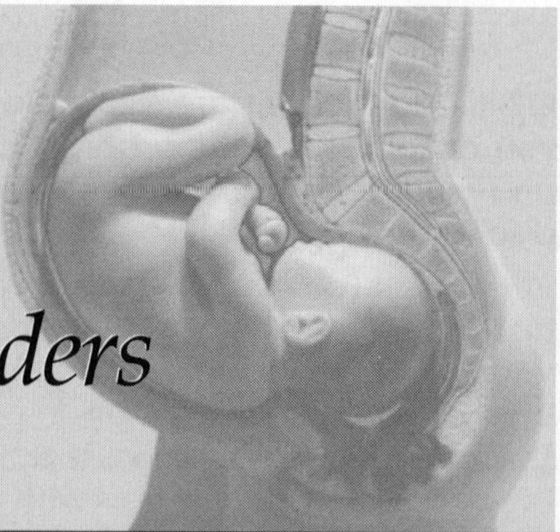

9 Menstrual Disorders and Menopause

CASE 9A PRIMARY AMENORRHEA: MULLERIAN AGENESIS (MRKH SYNDROME)

XYZ 18 year F
Unmarried
C/o Inablity to achieve menarche
No h/o Cyclical pain abdomen

Age of thelarche	11 years
Age of pubarche	10½ years

O/E
Ht – 5 ft
BMI – 25 kg/m^2

Secondary sexual characters–well developed

Breast development] Tanner stage 4
Pubic hair]

No skeletal deformity

P/A: No organomegaly or any lump felt

Q1. You have mentioned that the patient did not have cyclical pain abdomen. What would be your diagnosis if she did have a h/o cyclical pain abdomen?

If there is a history of cyclical pain abdomen associated with primary amenorrhoea, the diagnosis is cryptomenorrhoea, i.e. concealed menstruation due to obstructive lesion in the genital tract associated with functioning ovaries and endometrium. It could be due to imperforate hymen, transverse vaginal septum, or cervical agenesis/dysgenesis.

Q2. You have recorded that there was no lump on per abdomen examination. What would be the diagnostic implications had lump been present?

A lump in the abdomen may give the clue that it is *cryptomenorrhoea* (concealed menstruation) and the lump might be *hematometra* (collection of menstrual blood inside the uterine cavity). Sometimes the lump can be a pelvic kidney. A lump can also be ectopic testicles in abdomen, inguinal canal or labia in testicular feminization syndrome (androgen insensitivity syndrome). Lastly, a lump can be gonadoblastoma from dysgenetic gonads.

Q3. You have recorded that no adnexal mass was felt per rectum. What would be the diagnostic implications had an adnexal mass been felt on P/R?

P/R rules out cryptomenorrhoea by showing absence of palpable mass. Adnexal mass can be hematometra in rudimentary horn of uterus, ovarian endometriotic mass or tumor.

Q4. Why did you advise Hb and urine examination at an initial stage when these can be done later during PAC?

We can postpone it to next visit in this case. This is done in first visit to rule out disorders like anemia and diabetes.

Q5. You have recorded that the kidneys appear normal on USG. Why is an USG kidney important?

Renal abnormalities are associated in 20% of MRKH syndrome. Therefore USG examination is important to rule out single kidney, ectopic kidney, pelvic kidney, etc. before proceeding for vaginoplasty.

Q6. How many cases of Mayer Rockitansky Küster Hauser syndrome do you see in a month/year?

Not many, may be 12–14 cases per year, but since these cases are referred to us (at the tertiary hospital), it is important to diagnose them correctly and give timely advise.

Q7. What are the other causes of primary amenorrhea that are commoner than MRKH syndrome?

Three common causes of primary amenorrhoea in order of frequency are gonadal dysgenesis (50% Turner's syndrome), MRKH and androgen insensitivity syndrome (AIS).

Local examination:
External genitalia normal
Hymen patent
Blind vagina – length 2 cm from hymen

P/R: Cx and uterus not felt
No adnexal mass felt

Clinical diagnosis – Mullerian agenesis

Adv:
- Hb
- Urine (R & M)
- USG pelvis and abdomen for uterus and ovaries and kidneys
- Karyotype

Next visit
- Hb – 11g
- Urine NAD
- USG No uterus seen
- B/L ovaries normal
- B/L kidneys normal in shape, size and position
- Karyotype – 46XX

Δ Mullerian agenesis (Mayer Rockitansky Küster Hauser syndrome)

- Counselling to girl and parents regarding reproductive potential
- Vaginoplasty
- Investigations for PAC

Q8. How much delay in menarche constitutes primary amenorrhea? How would you diagnose it?

Primary amenorrhea is defined as absence of menarche by the age of 16 years with normal pubertal development or by age of 14 years without the onset of pubertal development. The history of illness and examination is of paramount importance in diagnosing it. History of cyclic pain abdomen suggests cryptomenorrhea. On examination one should note down sexual maturation, height and presence or absence of the Mullerian system (female genital tract–vagina, cervix, and uterus).

Complete Mullerian agenesis, as in this patient, calls for confirmation of findings by ultrasound. There are two possibilities and the diagnosis can be clinched only through karyotyping:

1. MRKH syndrome (46XX)
2. Androgen insensitivity syndrome (testicular feminizing syndrome) (46XY)

Q9. You mention AIS as one of the three main causes of primary amenorrhea. What is AIS?

In androgen insensitivity syndrome (AIS), earlier called the testicular feminizing syndrome, the patient is phenotypically female with male (46 XY) genotype and functional testes that secrete testosterone normally. It occurs due to the presence of abnormal androgen receptors that do not respond to testosterone. The internal genitalia are therefore neither male (since testosterone is ineffective) nor female (since MIS-Mullerian inhibiting substance is present). The external genitalia are female (since DHT is not formed) but the vagina ends blindly because there are no female internal genitalia. Individuals with this syndrome develop enlarged breasts at puberty and usually are considered to be normal women till they are diagnosed when they seek medical advice for absence of menarche. The patients are tall with no pubic, axillary or body hair and have well developed breasts.

Q10. Why is it important to differentiate MRKH from AIS if both the conditions, the treatment is vaginoplasty?

In AIS, the patient has functional testis which are mostly undescended. After the pubertal developement, gonadectomy is advised as testicular tumors can occur after this age in these patients. After gonadectomy ERT (estrogen replacement therapy) should be started.

Q11. How do you counsel the patients of primary amenorrhea when they want a baby?

The patient with MRKH syndrome does not have internal genitalia (tube, uterus and vagina) but has functional ovaries. Hence she does not menstruate but can mother a child with surrogacy, i.e. her ovum can be fertilized *in vitro* with her husband's sperm, and the embryo transferred to the surrogate mother's uterus. Also, they can have normal sexual life after vaginoplasty. The patient with AIS syndrome neither have a uterus, nor have functional ovaries. Therefore they neither menstruate nor can mother a child, even with surrogacy.

Flow Chart 9.1: Evaluation of primary amenorrhea

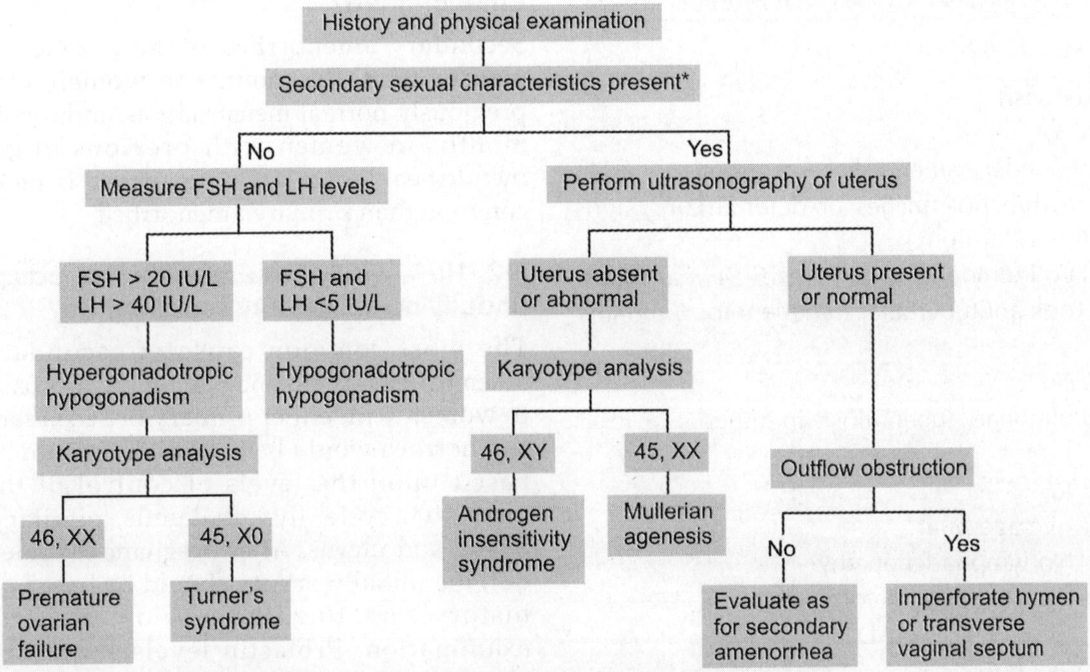

* Measure serum prolactin and thyroid functions. If diagnosed early, these are treatable

CASE 9B SECONDARY AMENORRHEA: TUBERCULAR ENDOMETRITIS

Mrs. X, 32 year

1st visit

C/o

secondary amenorrhea – 3 years

No h/o hot flushes or defeminizing signs (breast atrophy)

H/o Pulmonary tuberculosis 4 years back

Took antitubercular treatment for 6 months

H/o

Pulmonary tuberculosis in father

O/E

Average built

No lymphadenopathy

Breast – no galactorrhea

Chest, CVS – NAD

P/A NAD

P/S External genitalia, Cx, Vg, healthy

P/V Uterus R/V NS, B/L fornices free

Adv:

HMG with ESR

Mantoux test

S. prolactin & TFT

TVS on D2 of withdrawal bleeding for PCOS

X-ray chest PA view

R_x

1. Tab medroxyprogesterone acetate 10 mg × OD × 5 days
2. Watch for withdrawal bleeding for 7 days after stopping drug
3. Report after 14 days

2nd visit (after 2 weeks)

No withdrawal bleeding

Q1. The patient has reported with secondary amenorrhea. What is secondary amenorrhoea?

Secondary amenorrhea is the absence of menses for three months in women with previously normal menstruation, and for six months in women with previous oligomenorrhea. Secondary amenorrhea is more common than primary amenorrhea.

Q2. How would you identify the cause underlying secondary amenorrhea?

The most common cause of secondary amenorrhea is pregnancy. A logical approach to women with either primary or secondary amenorrhea would be to consider disorders based upon the levels of control of the menstrual cycle: hypothalamus, pituitary, ovary, and uterus. After pregnancy is ruled out, the initial work-up should be based on history and the findings on physical examination. Prolactin levels should be checked in most patients. The risk of amenorrhea is lower with subclinical hypothyroidism than with overt disease. However, the effects of subclinical hypothyroidism on menstruation and fertility are unclear, and abnormal thyroid hormone levels can affect prolactin levels. Hence, physicians should consider measuring thyroid-stimulating hormone (TSH) levels.

The progesterone challenge test is performed by giving a progestin: If the patient experiences withdrawal bleeding after the progestin medication is stopped then she has estrogen present but is not ovulating (anovulation). If no withdrawal bleeding occurs, either the patient has very low estrogen levels - or there is a problem with the outflow tract such as uterine synechiae (adhesions) or cervical stenosis (scarring). Further workup is done according to the algorithm.

Q3. You have recommended treatment as per DOTS guidelines. What are DOTS guidelines?

DOTS (Directly observed treatment, shortcourse) is recommended by WHO to improve compliance and ensure completion of ATT. Under DOTS strategy, every case of TB is categorized (according to the site, severity of disease, the bacterial load and the history of previous treatment) into one of the four categories (I-IV). In the context of genital TB, a new case with severe degree of affliction is allocated category I (highest priority) while less severe form is placed in category III. Category III is given four drugs in initial phase for 2 months and two drugs for 4 months in continuation phase (2HRZE + 4HR).

Patients with prior history of ATT are category II and require 5 drugs (HRZES) to be given in initial phase for 2 months and 3 drugs (HRE) in the continuation phase for 5 months. The total duration of therapy is 7 months.

S prolactin and TFT - normal
ESR 40 mm 1st hour
Mx – 10 × 10 mm

R_x
Sequential hormones
1. Tab premarin 0.625 mg × 1 OD × 21 days
2. Tab MPA 10 mg × OD 16th–25th day of starting Premarin
3. Wait for 7 days after stopping both the drugs

3rd visit

No withdrawal
Δ End organ failure
- Tubercular endometritis
- Asherman syndrome

Adv:
- Endometrial Bx for HPE, AFB smear, PCR, BACTEC culture

4th visit

EB for AFB
- BACTEC +ve AFB → treatment as per DOTS guidelines
  - BACTEC culture –ve → hysteroscopy for Asherman's syndrome and treatment at same sitting

Counselling regarding poor prognosis

Flow Chart 9.2: Evaluation of secondary amenorrhea

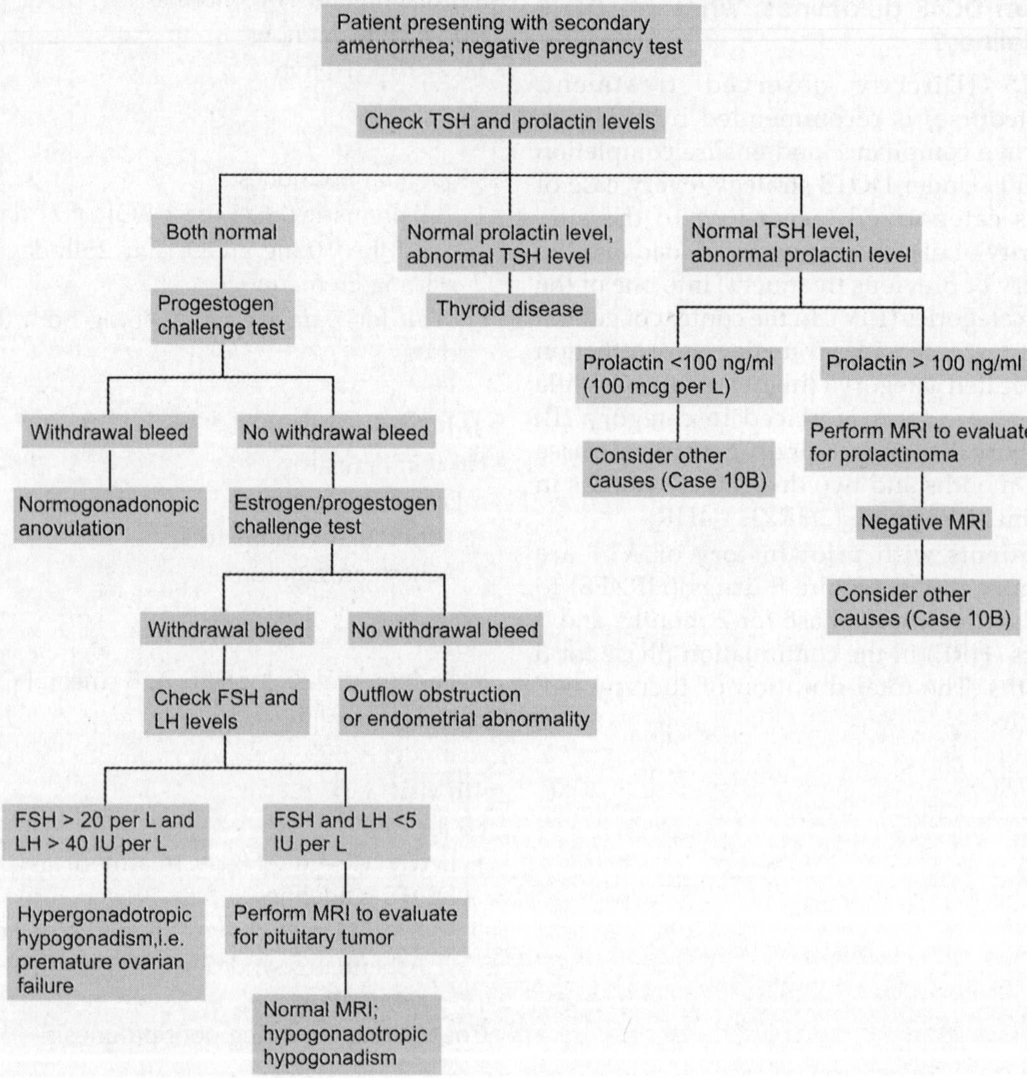

CASE 9C: MENORRHAGIA: DUB

1st visit 27.03.08

A 30- year-old female $P_{3+0+0+3}$

C/o menorrhagia – 2 years
No h/o dysmenorrhea

Past history
No h/o DM or HT or hormonal intake

M/H
LMP – 20.03.08
MC: 8–9 days/28 days
H/o passing clots

Ob/h
$P_{3+0+0+3}$
H/o laparoscopic tubal ligation 5 years back

O/E
Pallor +
Average built
Breast NAD
P/A NAD
P/S Cx and Vg healthy
P/v Ut R/v multiparous size
B/L fx free

Investigations:
1. HMG with platelet count
2. Urine (alb and sugar)
3. Coagulation profile,
4. TSH
5. TVS to look for myoma uterus, endometrial thickness and for ovaries.

2nd visit 4.04.08

All investigations—Normal

Δ DUB (Dysfunctional uterine bleeding)

Q1. The patient has presented with menorrhagia. What are the common causes of menorrhagia?

The common causes of menorrhagia are:

1. Pelvic pathology
   a. Fibroids
   b. Adenomyosis
   c. Pelvic infections
   d. Endometrial polyp
   e. IUCD
2. Dysfunctional uterine bleeding
3. Hypothyroidism
4. Coagulation disorder.

Q2. If DM, HT and hormonal intake are not among the common causes of menorrhagia, then why were their history elicited?

These are risk factors for endometrial malignancy and therefore history is taken in all cases of menorrhagia/menstrual disorders.

Q3. Does the h/o "laparoscopic tubal ligation 5 years back" give any diagnostic clue?

In a reproductive age group female presenting with abnormal uterine bleeding, it is important to consider pregnancy-related complications like abortion as a cause. Hence, a history of laparoscopic tubal ligation suggests that pregnancy is unlikely.

Q4. What led you to the diagnosis of DUB? What is AUB? Is it the same as DUB?

DUB is heavy and/or irregular menses in the absence of recognizable pelvic pathology, pregnancy or systemic bleeding disorder. In the present case no local pelvic pathology is found, the patient is not pregnant and no systemic disease is identifiable. Hence, the diagnosis of DUB is made.

AUB stands for abnormal uterine bleeding and is a better term to use for menstrual disorders. The diagnosis of DUB can change after investigations as in few cases there might be endometrial polyps, small myoma and tubercular endometritis. Otherwise in DUB,

Adv:
Combination of tab mefenamic acid 500 mg × 1 tds (antiprostaglandins) + tab tranexamic acid 500 mg 1 tds (antifibrinolytic drug) during periods for 3 months

Next visit
i. Patient is better → CST
ii. No improvement → Hysteroscopy and directed biopsy, or D&C if hysteroscopy is not available

the most common endometrial histology is normal endometrium which could be proliferative or secretary. In few cases there can be endometrial hyperplasia.

Q5. If the patient responds to medications, how long should be the CST?

Treatment is usually given for 3–6 months. After that see the menstrual pattern without treatment. In many cases cycles revert back to normal. If problem persists, treatment can be continued longer. If contraception is desired, combined oral contraceptive pills can be prescribed.

Q6. What is the usual course of events after the biopsy (by hysteroscopy) or D&C?

Benign conditions like endometrial polyps, or small submucus myoma if present, are removed during hysteroscopy or D&C. In such cases, the symptoms subside after the procedure. In DUB too, the removal of abnormal endometrium through D&C sometimes alleviates the symptoms. If symptoms persist or if the endometrial histology is abnormal, treatment is given according to the endometrial histology.

Q7. The algorithm shows that you recommend hormonal therapy to a menorrhagic patient with normal endometrium who neither responds to trenaxemic acid and antiprostaglandins, nor is aggreable to hysterectomy. What hormones do you prescribe to her?

In case of proliferative endometrium, progesterones for days 16–25 of the cycle (norethisterone 10 mg bd or medroxyprogesterone acetate 10 mg bd) or for 21 days of the cycle for 6 months can be prescribed. However, for secretory endometrium, combined pills can be used or short course of danazole (200 mg OD for 3 months) can be offered. In both types of endometrlum one can insert LNG-IUS (levonorgestrel intrauterine system-Mirena).

Q8. What is LNG-IUS. How does it Act?

The IUD with progestogen or intrauterine system (IUS) is a long acting reversible hormonal contraceptive device that is placed in the uterus. An IUS has a hormone cylinder that releases a progestin (a synthetic progestogen) called levonorgestrel. It releases 20 microgram LNG daily (LNG-20 IUS). It is effective for five years and useful contraceptive in perimenopausal period. This can also be used for menorrhagia and endometriosis as it causes endometrial atrophy and amenorrhoea in few cases. In some cases, use of an IUS may prevent a need for a hysterectomy.

Q9. The algorithm shows that your last resort in menorrhagic patients is hysterectormy or endometrial ablation. What is endometrial ablation?

The objective of endometrial ablation is complete destruction of the endometrium up to basal layer, resulting in amenorrhoea. In practice it is very difficult to achieve complete destruction and therefore only 20–30% of patients achieve amenorrhoea while the majority achieves oligomenorrhoea. The procedure is done with or without hysteroscopic guidance. Microwave or thermal ablation does not require the use of hysteroscope.

Flow Chart 9.3: Algorithm for management of menorrhagia

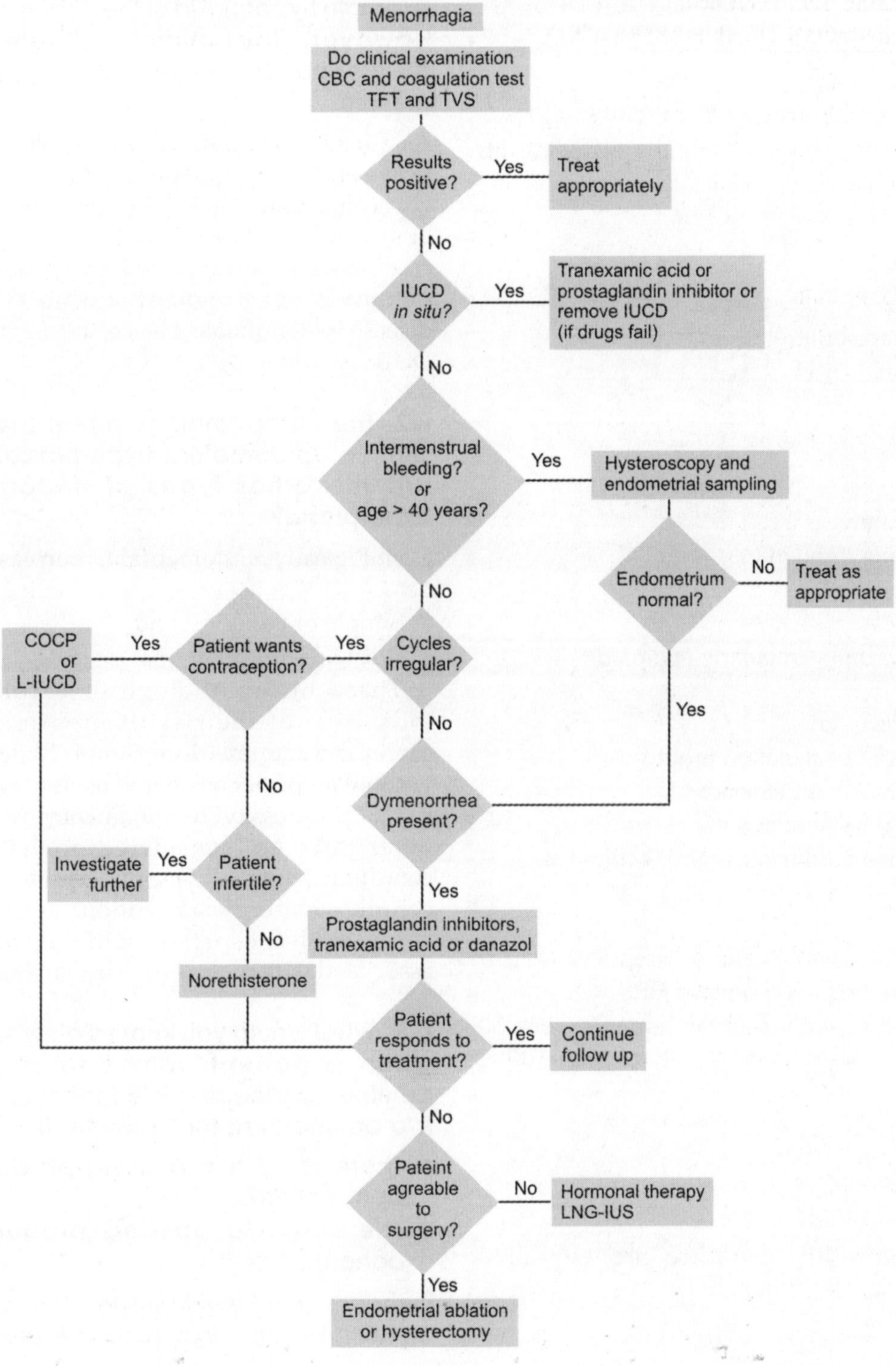

CASE 9D MENORRHAGIA: DUB ENDOMETRIAL HYPERPLASIA

45 years F $P_{4+0+0+4}$
C/o Continuous bleeding P/V – 1 month
H/o amenorrhea for 3 months preceding this
No h/o passing products of conception

O/E
GC fair
Pallor ++
Average built
Breast NAD

P/A NAD

P/s
Cx healthy
Bleeding through OS ++

P/v
Ut R/v, bulky, regularly enlarged

Investigations
CBC and coagulation profile
Urine – Alb and Sugar
TVS for uterine myoma,
Endometrial thickness and ovaries

Adv
→D & C after Hb and TVS report
→Curetting to be sent for HPE
→After D and C start tab norethisterone 10 mg × tds till bleeding stops, then 10 mg BD × 21 days

Next visit
TVS – normal
HPE – simple hyperplasia
- Counselling regarding progestational therapy for 9 months

Q1. The histopathology report of Case-9D is 'simple hyperplasia of the endometrium'. However, the clinical diagnosis is dysfunctional uterine bleeding. Please explain.

As already mentioned in case of 9C, DUB is heavy and/or irregular menses in the absence of recognizable pelvic pathology, pregnancy or systemic bleeding disorder. In the present case no local pelvic pathology is found, the patient is not pregnant and no systemic disease is identifiable. Hence, the diagnosis of DUB is made.

Q2. The histopathology report mentions 'Simple' endometrial hyperplasia. What are the other types of endometrial hyperplasia?

Histologically, endometrial hyperplasia may be:

a. Simple or complex, and
b. With or without atypia.

These histopathological features are indicative of the risk of progression to carcinoma endometrium. Simple hyperplasia without atypia is considered benign with <1% risk of progression to malignancy, while the other three are considered premalignant conditions. Simple hyperplasias with atypia, complex hyperplasia without atypia, and complex hyperplasia with atypia are associated with increasing risk of malignancy.

Q3. What would you immediately suspect when a patient comes to you with continuous bleeding P/V for 1 month and h/o amenorrhea for 3 months, if

a. There is no h/o passing products of conception?

b. There is h/o passing products of conception?

In the first case, I would suspect dysfunctional uterine bleeding (anovulatory) if pregnancy test is negative. In the second case, I would suspect incomplete abortion.

Q4. You have mentioned "progestational therapy for 9 months". What is it?

Progesterones for endometrial hyperplasia are effective when used in high doses (5 mg tid or 10 mg bid) between days 5 and 26 of the cycle out of 28. Either norethisterone or medroxy-progesterone acetate can be used. This has to be longterm therapy for 6–9 months.

- Same can be continued every cycle for 21 days with 7 days off drug × 6–9 cycle

Next visit

- Endometrium sampling after 9 months of therapy
- Endometrium reverts back to normal wait and watch the patient–she might enter normal menopause or can put LNG-IUS (levonorgestrel intrauterine system)

Q5. Why does the patient need counselling? Why do not you go for levonorgestrel IUS straight away?

Patient needs counseling for:

a. Adherence to therapy for 6–9 months, and
b. Reevaluation of endometrium after treatment.

Levonorgestrel IUCD, though very effective therapy for menorrhagia, is a costly device. Also, irregular bleeding is very common in the initial 3–4 months. Hence, proper counseling is important before insertion of LNG-IUS. In cases of Simple endometrial hyperplasia *without* atypia LNG-IUS can be inserted as the first line of therapy but oral medications are preferred for its lesser cost. However, simple hyperplasia *with* atypia is a precancerous lesion, and it is important to review the case after 6–9 months of progestogen therapy. Hence, oral medications are preferred.

Q6. What would be your management plan for endometrial hyperplasia that might be premalignant?

Simple hyperplasia without atypia is managed by hormonal therapy. Hyperplasia with atypia and complex hyperplasia are premalignant conditions and therefore hysterectomy is the right option for the patients of simple hyperplasia with atypia or complex hyperplasia. Very young patients who are infertile and desirous of pregnancy conservative therapy with progesterones are offered with stringent follow up.

CASE 9E FIBROID UTERUS

A 40-year-old female $P_{3+0+0+3}$
C/o
Heavy bleeding during periods–1 year
Cycles 8/30 days, previous cycles 3/30 days
H/o dysmenorrhoea present
No h/o intermenstrual bleeding and abnormal vaginal discharge

O/E
GC - fair
Pulse - 96/min;
BP: 120/80 mm/Hg
Pallor ++
Chest & CVS - NAD

P/A: NAD
P/S: Cervix and vagina - Normal
P/V: Ut - A/V, 12 weeks size; irregularly enlarged, mobile, Fornices are free
CI: Fibroid uterus (leiomyoma or myoma uterus)

Adv:
Hemoglobin
USG (TVS) for uterus and adenexa
Pap's smear

USG: Well circumscribed hypoechoic lesion in myometrium of anterior uterine wall suggestive of fibroid, endometrium normal. Both ovaries normal.

Pap's smear: Normal
Hb: 7 gm%

CI: Fibroid uterus with menorrhagia
Plan: Build up haemoglobin
Preop investigations
Hysterectomy

Q1. You have recorded that on P/V, the uterus was irregularly enlarged. What exactly is meant by "irregularly enlarged"? Do fibroids make the outer surface of the uterus irregular?

There are 3 general locations for fibroids:

1. Subserosal–on the outside surface of the uterus;
2. Intramural (commonest)- within the muscular wall of the uterus; and
3. Submucous (least common)- bulging in to the uterine cavity. The normal contour of the uterus is smooth. The subserosal fibroids bulge into the outer surface of the uterus and make it irregular.

Q2. Why is it necessary to ask for a history of intermenstrual bleeding in this case?

Intermenstrual bleeding raises suspicion of ulcerated/infected submucous fibroid or associated endometrial carcinoma.

Q3. Are there any alternatives to hysterectomy in the treatment of fibroids?

Yes, since the fibroid is an estrogen-dependent tumor, its growth can be checked by GnRH analogues, danazol, mifepristone (RU-486). However, the growth resumes after stopping the drug and therefore, the drug is used only preoperatively to buy time before surgery to improve the hemoglobin level. Surgical alternatives include **hysteroscopic resection** (removal of submucous fibroids using hysteroscope), myomectomy, and **uterine artery embolisation** (a method of shrinking the fibroids by cutting off their blood supply).

In this case, the patient has completed her family. Further managemant will depend on her desire to have menstrual function and her willingness to accept the risk of recurrence of menorrhagia and fibroids. Hysterectomy is the preferred treatment for her ailment.

Q1. What is differential diagnosis of this suprapubic mass?

In addition to uterine mass, midline suprapubic mass can be full bladder, an ovarian mass or non gynaecological mass. The latter is ruled out in this case by P/V examination. This mass is in continuity with cervix and therefore seems to be a uterine mass. A uniformly enlarged uterus associated with menorrhagia can be due to DUB, adenomyosis and fibroid uterus. In DUB and adenomyosis, the uterine enlargement is usually less than 12 weeks. Also, dysmenorr-hoea is very common in adenomyosis.

Q2. What is adenomyosis?

Adenomyosis is the presence of ectopic endometrial tissue within the myometrium. The patients have dysmenorrhea and menorrhagia. The dysmenorrhoea precedes the menses, remains throughout the cycle, and outlasts the cycle (triple dysmenorrhoea). The adenomyosis can be diffuse, or it may involve the uterus focally, creating an adenomyoma. With diffuse involvement, the uterus becomes bulky and heavier. Its diagnosis is clinical and aided by USG.

Q3. How is the obstetric history relevant in patients of fibroid?

The obstetric history and patient's desire to preserve future childbearing has important implications in the management. In the above-mentioned case one would like to conserve her fertility by retaining the uterus and not doing anything that impairs ovarian function.

Q4. You have noted that the patient had excessive bleeding "with clots". Does it make any difference if the bleeding is with or without clots?

Menorrhagia is defined when menstrual blood loss is >80 ml. It is difficult to assess the blood loss objectively. If patient has excessive

CASE 9F FIBROID UTERUS

A 22-year-old female
C/o Heavy period - 2 years.
M/H 5-7/28 d, excessive with clots, mild dysmenorrhoea +.

O/H Primary infertility, married for 3 yr

O/E
Pallor +
Thyroid and breast–normal
Systemic exam–normal

P/A
A firm well defined 14 weeks non-tender mass arising from pelvis, mobile
No ascites; Bowel sounds–normal

P/S Cervix, vagina–normal

P/V
Uterus enlarged to 14 weeks, firm regular, nontender, mobile, fornices free

P/R Rectal mucosa free
CI Fibroid (leiomyoma) uterus

Adv:
USG lower abdomen and pelvis
Hemoglobin,
Husband's semen analysis

Hb: 8 gm%
HSA: Normal
USG: 8 cm fibroid in posterior myo-metrium near fundus, endometrium normal, ovaries normal

Plan
Build up haemoglobin,
Transabdominal myomectomy with tubal assessment

bleeding or bleeds for > 7 days, it is clinically labelled as menorrhagia. Bleeding with clots indicates excessive bleeding. In normal menstrual cycle, menstrual blood is unclotted.

Q5. Why does fibroid cause menorrhagia?

Fibroids increase the surface area of endometrium. They are also associated with decreased uterine contractility, increased vascularity and sometimes associated endometrial hyperplasia.

Q6. How common is dysmenorrhea in patients of fibroid?

Dysmenorrhoea is a common associated symptom. Spasmodic dysmenorrhoea mostly occurs with submucous fibroids because uterus tries to expel it out. Congestive dysmenorrhoea can occur due to the size of the uterus and pelvic congestion.

Q7. Is the fibroid responsible for the patient's infertility?

Fibroids commonly do not affect the fertility. Occasionally submucous fibroids can interfere with the implantation, but all investigations of infertility should be normal in the couple before the fibroid is considered as the cause of infertility. In this case, the semen analysis is normal and the patient has not been fully investigated. She is being treated for fibroid because she is anemic due to the menorrhagia caused by the fibroid. At time of surgery it will be prudent to look for tubal patency so that she does not have to undergo tubal testing later.

Q8. Can a patient with a fibroid uterus become pregnant? Would there be any complication?

Yes, and the pregnancy is mostly uneventful though there is greater incidence of malpresentation, premature rupture of the membranes, placental abruption, and preterm birth, and greater risk of postpartum hemorrhage and uterine inversion (in case of large fundal fibroid). During pregnancy, the fibroids grow in size, become softer in consistency and merge with the uterus. When the fibroid degenerates during pregnancy and puerperium, it undergoes necrosis and suddenly becomes enlarged and painful (hence called *red degeneration*). The uterus is tender at the site of fibroid. The condition needs 'masterly inactivity', i.e. no surgical intervention. The patient needs to be nil orally, on intravenous fluids and rest.

Q9. How does myomectomy help the patient?

Myomectomy (enucleation of fibroid from its capsule and resuturing of the bed and reconstruction of the uterine surface) reduces menorrhagia. Heavy blood loss is a potential problem during myomectomy. Intramural fibroids less than 6 cm can be removed laparoscopically. Medical mangement is not effective.

Q10. Both Cases 9E and 9F are patients of fibroid uterus. What led you to different management plans for them?

The management of fibroid depends on factors like the age of patient, obstetric history, her desire to conserve menstrual function and the number, site and symptoms of the fibroid. Both the cases are of different age group and reproductive history with symptomatic leiomyoma. Both the cases need treatment but the approach and modality of the treatment are different.

Q1. How do you define menopause? This patient has amenorrhoea for only 8 months. Should she be diagnosed as menopausal?

Menopause is permanent cessation of menses due to decreasing ovarian function and marks the end of a woman's fertility. It is typically diagnosed after 12 months without a menstrual period. Although this patient has amenorrhea for just 8 months, she is symptomatic with lot of hot flushes and has a markedly raised FSH. This strongly supports the diagnosis of menopause though a definitive diagnosis can be made only after 12 months of amenorrhoea. Till then we can only say that the patient is in perimenopause.

Q2. What is the average age of menopause?

Menopause commonly occurs after 45 years of age. Average age of menopause is 51 years in the world. In India, it is around 47 years. When menopause occurs at an age of <40 years, it is referred as premature ovarian failure. At 42 years of age, it is early menopause but not premature.

Q3. You have recommended serum FSH to the patient. Is it essential to do serum FSH to prove diagnosis of menopause?

No, history and examination are adequate to diagnose menopause. One has to rule out causes of secondary amenorrhea and other conditions like depression, migraine and carcinoid syndrome that mimick menopausal symptoms. If women in menopausal age group have a history of irregular menses followed by its cessation with or without symptoms of estrogen deficiency and without any other abnormal findings, then no diagnostic tests are necessary to confirm menopause.

In this patient, FSH has been done to substantiate the diagnosis of menopause responsible for her symptoms because she is

CASE 9G MENOPAUSE

47 years, P_3L_3
C/o Amenorrhea – 8 months
Hot flushes + night sweats
Feeling depressed
No headache/visual disturbances
No past h/o depression

O/E
GPE – NAD, normotensive
Thyroid: Not enlarged
Breast – NAD, No galactorrhea

P/A NAD
P/S Cx, vagina healthy
P/V Cx ↑, Uterus R/V, normal size, mobile, B/L fornices–free, non-tender

CI – menopause

Adv:
- Urine for pregnancy test.

If negative
- Serum FSH

Next visit:
Serum FSH – 100 IU/L
Final diagnosis: Menopause

Plan:
- HRT (refer to specialist)
- Calcium supplementation

younger for age of menopause and is not yet amenorrhoeic for a year. Consistently elevated FSH levels (>40 IU) are diagnostic of menopause.

Q4. You have used the term 'menopausal symptoms'. What are these symptoms?

Common symptoms associated with menopause include hot flushes, night sweats, mood swings, vaginal dryness, decrease in sexual desire (libido), forgetfulness, insomnia and fatigue. These symptoms can be seen during perimenopause (years of menopausal transition) along with menstrual irregularity.

Q5. Till what age has successful pregnancy been reported? Till what age would you advise pregnancy test? Would you advise pregnancy test as a routine even if the patient feels that pregnancy is unlikely?

The latest age by which successful pregnancy by spontaneous conception has been reported is 59 years, but the world's oldest mother gave birth to a child just before her 67th birthday, she had conceived via IVF.

One can be sure of menopause only when menses have ceased for 12 months. The preceding period during which menstrual cycles become abnormal is known as perimenopause. This period can be 5–6 years long. Conception is possible during perimenopause. Though in this age group fertility decreases markedly, pregnancy should still be ruled out if effective contraception is not being used. Pregnancy is unlikely after 1 year of the last menstruation.

Q6. If pregnancy can occur till such late age then how long contraception should be given?

As infrequent ovulation can occur rarely after last menstruation, it is recommended that in women under 50, contraception should be continued for two years after last menstruation. In women over 50, contraception should be continued for one year after last menstruation. These are Western recommendations: May be we can take 45 years as the cut off age since menopause occurs early in our population.

Q7. On examination, you have recorded that there is no galactorrhea. Why do you look for galactorrhea?

Hyperprolactinemia is an important cause of secondary amenorrhoea requiring further investigations. Hence we look for galactorrhoea which is a sign of hyperprolactinemia (discussed in chapter 10 on infertility).

Q8. In this case, history alone seems to be enough for diagnosing the patient. Why do we need to examine her?

Though history is highly suggestive of menopause, examination is still done to rule out any other cause of secondary amenorrhoea and other symptoms. In this age group, a complete examination also gives an opportunity to screen for other health problems including malignancies and premalignant conditions.

Q9. What is HRT?

HRT is Hormone Replacement Therapy also known as Estrogen Replacement Therapy (ERT). The purpose is to replace the ovarian hormones (Estrogen) which are decreased due to loss of ovarian activity. In HRT Estrogens are given (along with progestogen if uterus is intact). Estrogens can be given via oral, transdermal route for systemic actions or vaginal route for local effects on vaginal epithelium.

Q10. Is hormone replacement therapy advisable in all menopausal women?

No, HRT is prescribed when menopause is associated with severe vasomotor symptoms (hot flashes, night sweats and mood swings and sleep disturbaces caused by these) and urogenital symptoms (vaginal dryness, dyspareunia, urinary symptoms). In vaginal atrophy, estrogen cream is prescribed for intravaginal application. HRT is also prescribed till the normal age of menopause in premature menopause (including surgical ones).

Oral estrogens with/without progestogens are prescribed usng the lowest dose of estrogens for the shortest period required by the patient. The contraindications to HRT are roughly the same as those for oral contraceptive use.

Q11. You have prescribed calcium supplementation. Should calcium be routinely recommended in postmenopausal women?

A postmenopausal woman should take 1200 mg of elemental calcium along with 400 IU of Vit D daily. The dietary intake should be increased but oral supplementation is often required lifelong, more so in women who have high risk for osteoporosis. In the present case, she had early menopause, so calcium supplementation is very important.

Q12. Can HRT be taken by the patient over the counter without prescription?

No, due to its potentially harmful effects, HRT should be supervised by a trained specialist. HRT increases the risk of endometrial cancer (if estrogen is given without progestogen), breast cancer, thromboembolism and stroke.

10 *Infertility*

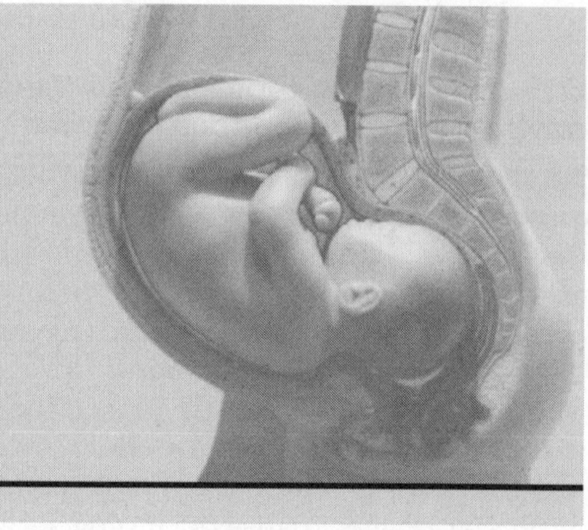

CASE 10A (MALE INFERTILITY)

ABCDEF 23-year F

1st visit 28.2.08

C/o

Inability to conceive 4 years

No h/o coital problems

Husband works in government job and is nonsmoker and nonalcoholic

M/H

LMP 14.02.08

MC–4/28 days, Regular cycles

O/E Thyroid – Not enlarged

Breast – No galactorrhea

P/A NAD

P/S Cx and Vg healthy

P/V Ut R/V, normal size,
B/L fx free

Investigations

- HSA (Husband's semen analysis)
- Hmg with ESR
- Urine alb, Sugar
- VDRL
- TVS (Transvaginal sonography) from Day 9 of the cycle for follicular monitoring

Q1. After how many years of inability to conceive is a couple called infertile? What are the common causes of infertility?

Infertility is usually defined as the inability to conceive after one year of unprotected intercourse. This condition may further be classified as primary infertility, in which no previous pregnancies have occurred, and secondary infertility, in which a prior pregnancy (irrespective of the outcome) has occurred. The diagnosis of infertility often comes in two stages, the first stage being the general infertility diagnosis, and the second stage being a diagnosis of the specific cause of the infertility. Infertility is almost a symptom itself.

Two of the most common causes of female infertility are ovulatory dysfunctions and tubal or peritoneal factors. The two common causes of male infertility are oligospermia (this is the most common cause of male factor infertility) and sperm abnormalities (malformed sperm or low motility).

Q2. What are the criteria of abnormal semen?

If there is deviation from reference values as per WHO criteria, it is labelled as abnormal semen. These values are referred as reference values because these are not the absolute minimum requirement to achieve a pregnancy. But, values outside the reference range suggest a male infertility factor that may require additional clinical/laboratory evaluation.

Normal reference values for Semen Analysis (WHO 2002)

Parameter	*Reference value*
Volume	2 ml or more
pH	7.2 or more
Sperm concentration	$>20 \times 10^6$/ml
Total sperm number	$>40 \times 10^6$
Motility	>50% with progressive motility
Morphology	>15% normal (strict criteria)*
Round cells	<5 million/ml
White blood cells	<1 million/ml
Sperm agglutination	< 2 (on a scale of 2–3)

* Data from assisted reproduction suggest that fertilization rates drop if sperm morphology falls below 15% of the normal forms using strict criteria to assess sperm morphology. Using this system, the entire spermatozoon–including the head, midpiece and tail is assessed and even mild abnormalities are classified as abnormal.

Q3. The table on semen analysis refers to round cells. What are round cells?

Round cells detected in semen can be either white blood cells (lymphocytes) or immature germ cells. These two cells can be distinguished by an immunoperoxidase – staining technique that identifies leukocytes. The presence of immature germ cells in the semen signifies a defect in spermatogenesis, while an abnormal number of WBCs suggests genital tract infection or inflammation.

Q4. Is semen analysis done in all case of infertility?

Yes, abnormalities in the male are the sole cause of infertility in approximately 20% of

Adv:
- Review with investigations
- Explained about fertile period

2nd visit 05.03.08

Husband's semen analysis:

Azoospermia or severe sperm abnormality

Adv
- Examination of male partner
- Repeat semen examination

3rd visit 12.03.08

Examination of male partner: Look for

GPE

Level of masculinization

Stigmata of chromosomal anomaly

Gynecomastia

Inguinal hernia or relevant surgical scars

Genital examination:

Varicocele or any scrotal swelling

Undescended testis

Epididymis or vas deferens:

Nodularity

Tenderness

Testicular volume, sensation, consistency

Examination Normal

4th visit 20.03.08

Repeat semen analysis result:

Abnormality:

Asthenospermia → check antibodies

Azoospermia or severe oligospermia ($<5 \times 10^6$ per ejaculate)

Adv:

S. FSH and S. testosterone

5th visit 01.04.08

Δ (depending on S.FSH and S.testosterone)

Both normal: Obstructive cause

Raised FSH, normal/low testosterone: Primary testicular failure

Low FSH, low testosterone: Hypogonadotrophic hypogonadism

Treatment

1. Primary testicular failure → Artificial insemination of donor semen/adoption
2. Obstructive cause: Vasogram → microsurgery or sperm aspiration and ICSI (Intracytoplasmic sperm insemination)
3. Hypogonadotrophic hypogonadism → treat with gonadotropins

the infertile couples and are an important contributing factor in another 20–40% of the couples with reproductive failure. By single non-invasive test (semen analysis) one can rule out male factor, therefore it is done before investigation the female partner with invasive tests.

Q5. You have recorded that the husband is nonsmoker and nonalcoholic. Are smoking and alcoholism known causes of infertility?

These decrease the semen quality.

Q6. What is the relevance of husband's occupational history in infertility (c.f., husband works in government job)? The stress factor?

Is not related to stress. Hot climate for testis, e.g. drivers, people working in hot furnaces in factories, results in impaired spermatogenesis.

Q7. What is the relevance of galactorrhea in infertility?

Clinical examination for galactorrhoea should be done in all cases of infertility to rule out hyperprolactinemia, which is a known cause of infertility (discussed in case of hyperprolactinemia).

Q8. What type of clues to the cause of infertility might be provided by P/A, P/S or P/V examination?

These will rule out anatomical defect of genital tract, and genital infections (acute or chronic).

Q9. Among the investigations, semen analysis and VDRL are understandable. But how are hemogram with ESR and urine test relevant to the investigation of infertility? (TB and DM?)

Hemogram and urine test are done as routine to rule out major medical illnesses and provide baseline investigations for further workup of the female partner. ESR is done to know chronic infection, if this high >20 or there is history s/o TB, X-ray chest is ordered.

Q10. What is "TVS from D9 for follicular monitoring"?

This is USG (preferable transvaginal) examination to document follicular development and ovulation. This is one of the tests for ovulation in which serial ultrasounds are done from day 9 of the menstrual cycle taking LMP as D1.

Q11. Who does the semen analysis? Pathology lab? Who does the examination of the male partner? Physician? Surgeon?

Pathology lab. Ideally the semen sample should be collected by masturbation into a clean container. Two to three days abstinence is advised before the test to have better quality semen. If possible, semen sample should be collected in a private room within or near the laboratory. If it is not possible, the specimen can be collected at home but should be kept at body temperature during transportation. It should not be collected in condom as this might contain spermicides. Regardless of the method of collection, the semen sample should be examined within 1 hour after collection. Ideally the doctor taking history and examination at infertility clinic should also do the examination of male partner. Gross abnormalities in semen are an indication for thorough evaluation of the male partner by a urologist or a surgeon.

Q12. What antibodies do you check for in asthenospermia?

Elevated levels of antisperm antibodies in the male have been associated with impairment of fertility. Since spermatozoa mature after immunologic tolerance has been established, unique antigens are expressed on their surfaces, but the sperm are normally shielded from an immune response by the blood-testis barrier. Any event that disrupts the continuity of the male reproductive tract will increase the risk of formation of antisperm antibodies. This often occurs in cases of ductal obstruction, previous genital infection, testicular torsion or trauma and sterilization reversal.

Though routine screening for antisperm antibodies is not clinically useful, marked sperm clumping or agglutination or isolated asthenospermia can signal the presence of antisperm antibodies. Most widely used tests for detection of antisperm antibodies involve the bead or latex particles with attached antibodies (against human immunoglobulins IgG and IgA) that bind to antibodies on the surface of sperms. The sperm suspension is mixed with a suspension of immunobeads. Preparation is examined under phase contrast microscopy. Immunobeads adhere to the motile spermatozoa that have surface antibodies and the percentage of these is counted.

Q13. What is the treatment for male infertility and asthenospermia?

Treatment options for male infertility most commonly involve techniques of assisted reproduction, including IUI (intrauterine insemination) or IVF (in vitro fertilization). If the sperm count is very low, ICSI (intracytoplasmic sperm injection), wherein a single sperm is injected into each egg, may be used with IVF. If no motile sperms are observed, a sperm viability test is performed to differentiate the viable nonmotile sperms from the dead sperms. The viable sperms are then used for ICSI. In certain cases, sperm is aspirated directly from the epididymis or testicle and accordingly, the techniques are called MESA (microsurgical epididymal sperm aspiration) or PESA (percutaneous epididymal sperm aspiration), TESE (testicular sperm extraction), and TESA (testicular sperm aspiration). When large varicoceles are present, surgical intervention to remove the varicocele may result in improved fertility. Fertility drugs such as clomid, FSH or hCG may be applicable in certain cases (Table 10.1).

Treatment of asthenospermia/antisperm antibodies is intrauterine insemination with washed sperms after semen preparation or IVF-ET with prepared semen. Advances in assisted reproductive techniques has replaced the use of high dose steroids in cases of antisperm antibodies.

Q14. Is IUI done in our hospital? How is it done?

Yes, IUI (intrauterine insemination) is done in our hospital. The semen from the male partner or a donor are washed and the motile sperms in it are separated from the seminal plasma, dead sperms, debris and leucocytes. The

Table 10.1: Treatment for male infertility

Management	*Condition/ abnormality*	*Specific treatment*
Medical	Hypogonadotrophic hypogonadism	Gonadotropins
	Symptomatic genital tract infections	Antibiotics
	Idiopathic oligo/astheno/teratospermia	Empirical treatment with antiestrogens (clomiphene, tamoxifen)/ Gonadotropins/androgens
Surgical	Obstructive azoospermia Obstruction in vas deferens (including sterilization procedure)	Microsurgical vasovasostomy or vasoepididymostomy
	Ejaculatory duct obstruction	Transurethral resection of the obstruction
	Varicoceles with semen abnormalities	Varicocele repair
Artificial insemination	Mild to moderate oligospermia Asthenospermia Low ejaculate volume Antisperm antibodies Hypospadias Retrograde ejaculation Neurological impotence Sexual dysfunction	Intrauterine insemination (IUI) with or without ovulation induction
	Unexplained infertility	Intrauterine insemination with ovarian stimulation
Assisted reproductive technologies (ART)	Severe oligo/astheno/teratozoospermia	IVF and ICSI
	When IUI is unsuccesful	IVF, ICSI
	Obstructive azoospermia (uncorrectable obstruction or congenital absence of vas)	Epididymal sperm aspiration (MESA or PESA) and ICSI
	Obstructive azoospermia in which epididymal sperm aspiration fails	Testicular sperm aspiration/ exraction (TESA/ TESE) and ICSI
Artificial insemination with donor semen	Non-obstructive azoospermia All the conditions mentioned in ART, if ART is not desirable or affordable	IUI with donor sperm

prepared semen is introduced via a intrauterine catheter in the uterine cavity during the time of ovulation so as to increase the chances of conception. Hence, it is also important to monitor the time of ovulation. IUI can be combined with *controlled ovarian stimulation* whereby ovulation is induced by giving Comiphene 100 mg OD × 5 days. Follicular monitoring is done and when mature follicle reaches the size of 20–24 mm, Inj hCG is given for ovulation trigger and IUI is done 36 hours after hCG injection.

IUI is not to be confused with more complex types of ART (assisted reproductive techniques) like IVF–ET (*in vivo fertilization and embryo transfer*) or ICSI (*intracytoplasmic sperm injection*) which involves manipulation of oocytes outside the body. IVF is indicated when very few motile sperms are retrievable or pregnancy is not possible due to associated tubal block.

Q1. Is MRI done in all cases of hyperprolactinemia?

Purpose of doing MRI is to rule out macroadenoma (>1 cm) of the pituitary. Although MRI will detect both micro- as well as macroadenoma, it is *not* important to know the presence of microadenoma because:

i. Its treatment is invariably medical, and
ii. It does not grow during pregnancy and therefore no treatment is needed during pregnancy.

MRI is ordered when any of the following is present

a. Serum prolactin is >100 ng/ml
b. X-ray skull shows enlarged sella turcica
c. Presence of visual symptoms or headache

Q2. Is it important to stop bromocriptine during pregnancy?

Bromocriptine is not a teratogenic drug and therefore it is continued during pregnancy in patients with macroadenoma. However, in patients of microadenoma, there is no need to continue it during pregnancy.

Q3. Can we use any other drug instead of bromocriptine?

Cabergoline is a better tolerated drug and is longer acting, therefore is used once a week. Bromocriptine is preferred over it in cases of infertility as the teratogenic potential of cabergoline is not yet known.

Q4. Besides hyperprolactinemia, are there other types of hormonal imbalances (estrogen, progesterone, etc.) that are associated with (1) hypomenorrhea or (2) infertility?

Will discuss in different causes of anovulation, e.g. PCOS.

CASE 10B FEMALE INFERTILITY: ANOVULATION (HYPERPROLACTINEMIA)

ABCDEF 23-year F

1st visit 28.02.08

C/o

Inability to conceive 4 years
Delayed cycles with hypomenorrhoea 2 years. MC–2/45 days
No h/o coital problems
Husband works in government job and is nonsmoker and nonalcoholic

M/H

LMP 24.02.08

O/E

Thyroid – Not enlarged
Breast – B/L galactorrhea +
P/A NAD
P/S Cx and Vg healthy
P/V Ut R/V, normal size, fx free

Investigations:

- Husband's semen analysis
- Hmg with ESR
- Urine: Albumin and Sugar
- VDRL
- Serum prolactin
- TSH

Adv:

Review with investigations
Explained about fertility period

2nd visit 05.03.08

Semen analysis and all other investigations-normal
S prolactin – 200 ng/ml

Adv:

Ask for headache and visual symptoms

- Evaluate the woman for drug intake (antidepressants, alpha methyl dopa, metoclopramide)
- Thyroid function and kidney function tests.

If No h/o drug intake

MRI brain for imaging pituitary gland

3rd visit 09.03.08

TFT and KFT–noraml

MRI –pituitary microadenoma

T/t tab bromocriptine 2.5 mg at bed time after meals

Can be increased to one tab twice a day after a week up to maximum of three tabs

4th visit 30.03.08

Had normal period

LMP 28.03.03

Adv:

Continue bromocriptine and stop it as soon as pregnancy is confirmed.

Q5. How hyperprolactinemia is associated with infertility?

Hyperprolactinemia inhibits the pulsatile release of GnRH. It also inhibits progesterone synthesis by corpus luteum resulting in luteal phase defects (LPD). Therefore it can be associated with oligomenorrhoea, amenorrhoea, dysfunctional uterine bleeding, LPD, infertility, hirsutism and osteoporosis. The infertility is due to ovulatory dysfunction, i.e. oligo or anovulation and LPD.

Q6. Is hypomenorrhea associated with infertility?

This will depend on the cause of hypomenorrhoea. If latter is due to hyperprolactinemia or endometrial tuberculosis, then answer is yes.

Q7. Can galactorrhea occur in the absence of hyperprolactinemia?

There are two types of clinical situations

- *Hyperprolactinemia without galactorrhoea:* For galactorrhea to occur in hyperprolactinemia, oestrogenised breast is prerequisite. Males do not experience galactorrhoea in hyperprolactinemia. In females only 33% of women with hyperprolactinemia have galactorrhea because of associated hypoestrogenic state or heterogeneity of prolactin molecule, i.e high circulating level of prolactin may not represent material capable of interacting with breast receptors.
  Prolactin circulates in three molecular sizes: little, big and big big. The most of the biological activity is due to little form, the big forms are usually immunoreactive but have weak biological activity. Therefore it may be that high circulating level of prolactin is basically big big molecule which is biologically less active.
- *Galactorrhea without hyperprolactinemia*: On the other hand galactorrhea can be seen in women with normal serum prolactin. This can be explained by one of the 4 mechanisms:
  1. There can be increased sensitivity of the breast receptors to normal prolactin levels.
  2. It may be due to intermittent prolactin elevation.
  3. It may be due to excess sleep induced prolactin pulses.
  4. May be due to an elevated biologically active prolactin which is not immuno reactive.

Q8. What is the normal range of S. prolactin?

0–20 ng/ml

Q9. What causes hyperprolactinemia - hypothyroidism, hyperthyroidism, or both?

Primary hypothyroidism results in increase in TRH which stimulates prolactin release. In fact, hypothyroidism is the cause of hyperprolactinemia in 5–10% of cases. For hyperprolactinemia it is important to rule out primary hypothyroidism, as this condition is treatable.

Q10. What causes infertility in hyperprolactinemia?

Hyperprolactinemia results in infertility due to disorders of ovulation. Increased prolactin due to any cause leads to suppression of pulsatile release of GnRH and also decreases the ovarian responsiveness to gonadotropin hormones thus disturbing ovulation.

Q11. Why do we get a KFT done?

Serum prolactin is excreted thru kidneys. In cases of deranged KFT there can be hyperprolactinemia.

Q12. Why must we do a MRI to look for a microadenoma when the prolactin levels alone can establish the cause of infertility? Conversely, can hyperprolactinemia occur in the absence of radiographically detectable micro- or macro-adenoma?

MRI in this case is essential to rule out *macro- (not micro-adenoma)* since with a prolactin level of 200 ng/ml it is quite possible that pituitary gland might be harboring macroadenoma. Hyperprolactinemia can occur due to various other causes but often the levels are <100 ng/ml.

Q13. What are the commonest causes of female infertility?

Among female factors, tubal and ovulatory causes are the commonest followed by endometriosis.

Q14. What is follicular monitoring and how is it done?

Follicular development and ovulation can be visualized by serial ultrasonography. In a spontaneous normal cycle, a cohort of follicles is recruited in early follicular phase from pool of primordial follicles. Under the influence of endogenous FSH, few follicles start secreting estrogen and continue to grow till these attain an average size of 20–24 mm and then ovulation occurs. These changes are observed by ultrasonography, preferably transvaginal USG. This is known as follicular monitoring. Monitoring, usually done on alternate days, starts on day 8 or 9 of the menstrual cycle. Usually one or two follicles grow at the rate of 2 mm/day. The growing follicles are identified up at 8–10 mm diameter and followed up till it reach the size of 20–24 mm. Intrafollicular echoes start appearing when the follicle is mature. A completely echo free follicle is not a good sign. After ovulation, the follicle becomes smaller and its wall becomes irregular, filling with low levels of echoes.

Q15. What are the tests for ovulation?

Commercially available kits can detect the urinary LH surge that coincides with ovulation, or the serum progesterone surge that coincides with the mid-leuteal phase. Due to cost constraints, these tests are not done at our center. Ultrasonic follicular monitoring is a non-invasive method to monitor follicle growth, detect ovulation and monitor ovulation induction. The basal body temperature remains the cheapest way to detect ovulation. Although an invasive procudure, premenstrual EB (endometrial biopsy) is widely used in India as a test for ovulation because it also helps in diagnosing tuberculosis (which is widely prevalent in India) and luteal phase defects.

CASE 10C OVULATORY DYSFUNCTION

ABCDEF 23-year F

1st visit

C/o

Inability to conceive 4 years

Delayed cycles 2 years

No h/o coital problems

Husband works in job and is nonsmoker and nonalcoholic

M/H

H/o delayed cycles +

3–4 /40–45 days, normal flow

LMP 24.02.08

O/E

Obesity +, BMI - 32

No evidence of hirsutism

Thyroid – Not enlarged

Breast – no galactorrhoea

P/A NAD

P/S Cx and Vg healthy

P/V Ut R/V normal size, B/L fornices free

Investigations

- D2 USG for ovaries to rule out PCOS
- HSA
- HMG with ESR
- Urine alb, Sugar
- VDRL
- Serum prolactin, S. TSH
- Follicular monitoring from D 9

Adv:

- Review with investigations
- Explained about fertile period

Q1. You have advised ovulation induction with clomiphene. What is its procedure?

Clomiphene is given 50 mg tablet OD × 5 days starting from D3 of cycle. Follicular monitoring is not mandatory but should be done to know whether ovulation has occurred or not. The dose of clomiphene can be increased to 100 mg and still further 150 mg OD × 5 days till ovulation is achieved. With ovulatory dose, one carries on with 3 cycles before switching on to other ovulation inducing agents.

Q2. What is PCOS (polycystic ovarian syndrome)?

Women with at least two of the following criteria are said to have PCOS:

i. Evidence of hyperandrogenism, biochemical or clinical in the absence of non-clasical adrenal hyperplasia. Most commonly, hirsutism, acne and crown pattern baldness.

ii. Ovulatory dysfunction, amenorrhea or oligomenorrhea.

iii. Morphological polycystic ovary (PCO) on ultrasound (even single PCO is considered as part of the syndrome.

Q3. What is PCO (polycystic ovary)?

USG is the gold standard for diagnosis of PCO. For diagosis of PCO, USG (TVS) is done on Day 2 of menstrual cycle. The diagnostic criteria are:

1. Presence of 12 or more follicles of 2–9 mm
2. Ovarian volume 12 ml or more.
3. Bright echogenic stroma.

PCO in the absence of clinical symptoms does not have any clinical relevance.

Q4. How do you diagnose insulin resistance (IR)?

Insulin resistence is reduced glucose response to insulin. This leads to hyperinsulinemia as a compensatory mechanism. Fasting serum insulin levels are with upper limit of 10–20 U/ml in various labs. Level greater than this indicates insulin resistance. One can do S.fasting glucose to insulin ratio, <4.5 indicates insulin resistance. Another alternative test is 2 hour glucose level after 75 g glucose intake on fasting stomach.

	Plasma Glucose
Normal level	<140 mg%
Impaired	140–199 mg%
NIDDM	200 mg% or higher

One should assume that all obese women with PCOS have insulin resistance because considerable overlap in insulin levels between normal women and patients with PCOS and anovulation. Non-obese women can also have insulin resistance. Therefore IR should be tested in all women with PCOS.

Q5. How are the other causes of anovulation managed?

In all cases of ovulatory dysfunction, thyroid disorders and hyperprolactinemia should be ruled out or treated if present. PCOS is ruled out next. Thereafter, the day 2/3 FSH, LH is estimated to differentiate between hypothalamic or ovarian disorders. In hypogonadotrophic hypogonadism (a hypothalamic disorders), pulsatile GnRH or daily injections of gonadotropins are used to induce ovulation. Hypothalamic disorders can also be due to excessive stress and should be managed with psychiatrist consultation. Ovarian failure or resistant ovary syndrome do not respond to ovulation induction and oocyte donation is the answer.

2nd visit

Semen analysis and all other investigations–normal

D 2 USG shows **polycystic ovaries** (PCO)

Follicular monitoring– anovulation

Investigations: Fasting S. insulin and glucose

Tubal patency testing by HSG

Adv.

Weight reduction

Lifestyle modification

3rd visit

HSG → B/L tubes patent

No insulin resistance

Adv:

Ovulation induction with clomiphene

Insulin resistance +ve →

S.insulin ↑ed

Or

F.insulin/F glucose ratio <4.5

Adv:

Tab metformin 500 tds

(Start metformin 500 mg OD on week 1, then BD on week 2 and tds from week 3 onwards for 6–12 months)

(Baseline LFT and KFT should be normal)

4th visit

No pregnancy in 6 months → add clomiphene for 6 cycles → no pregnancy → consider gonadotrophins or ovarian drilling.

Pregnancy confirmed → stop metformin

CASE 10D FEMALE INFERTILITY: TUBAL BLOCK

ABCDEF 23 year F

1st visit 28.02.08

C/o

Inability to conceive 4 years
Regular cycles with hypomenorrhoea 2 yrs
No h/o coital problems
Husband works in job and is nonsmoker and nonalcoholic

M/H

LMP 24.02.08

O/E

Thyroid – Not enlarged
Breast – no galactorrhea
P/A NAD
P/S Cx and Vg healthy
P/V Ut R/V normal size fx free

Investigations

- Husband's semen analysis
- HMG with ESR
- Urine alb, Sugar
- VDRL
- Serum prolactin, TSH

Adv:

- Review with investigations
- Explained about fertility period

2nd visit 05.03.08

Semen analysis and all other investigations–normal
S prolactin, TSH – normal
Endometrial biopsy in premenstrual phase for histopathology and AFB smear and culture

3rd visit 09.05.08

EB - secretory endometrium, No AFB
Adv: HSG (Hysterosalpingography) in post-menstrual phase (within 10 days of LMP)

Q1. Why is HSG done within 10 days of ovulation? How is it done?

HSG is done in postmenstrual phase to be sure that patient is not pregnant and before the next ovulation to avoid any radiation hazards. Under fluoroscopic guidance, Conray 420 (a water soluble iodine based dye) is injected trans cervically through Leech Wilkinson's cannula or foley's catheter. Sequential films are taken to trace the path of dye into the peritoneal cavity.

Q2. When tubal block has been diagnosed in this case then why do you go for laparoscopy?

HSG is a simple OPD procedure which is used as a screening test for tubal patency. Even when HSG demonstrates patency, there is still a little chance (~5%) that the tube is occluded. If HSG reveals obstruction, there is still a relatively high chance (~60%) that the tube is open. Therefore when HSG shows tubal block, it needs to be confirmed through diagnostic laparoscopy in which dilute methylene blue dye is injected in the uterus through cervical canula (chromo-tubation). Tubal patency is indicated by the flowing out of dye from fimbrial ends. The advantage of laparoscopy is that any peritoneal cause of infertility, e.g. endometriosis, PID, previous ectopic pregnancy and tuberculosis can be detected simultaneously. Tuboplasty can also be performed at the same time if possible.

Another test to check tubal patency is SIS (Saline infusion sonography). In TVS (transvaginal sonography) with saline infusion, saline is injected into the uterine cavity through a Foley's catheter. The collection of fluid in the pelvic cavity during the procedure confirms that at least one tube is patent. Its disadvantage is that it can detect only a bilateral tubal block. SIS can be done as an alternative to HSG but final confirmation is by laparoscopy.

Q3. How do you ascertain whether tubal block is because of tubercular or non-tubercular infection?

Various findings on laparoscopy may suggest genital tuberculosis. Laparoscopic findings are tubercles on the peritoneal surfaces, tubes or ovaries, caseous nodules, peritoneal adhesions, b/l tubo-ovarian masses, thick rigid tubes, beaded tubes, encysted ascites, tobacco-pouch appearance of the tubes, b/l cornual block, multiple site blocks of the tubes. Such findings if present will suggest tuberculosis as the likely cause of genital tuberculosis.

Q4. Why is EB done in this case?

The hypomenorrhoea of the patient can be due to endometrial tuberculosis, which is highly prevalent in India. The EB is done to diagnose endometrial tuberculosis. If genital tuberculosis is suspected, HSG test can lead to a flare up of the tubercular infection. Therefore before doing HSG, it is important to rule out endometrial tuberculosis when clinical suspicion is high, as in the present case.

Q5. Do we get any more information from endometrial biopsy other than diagnosis of tuberculosis?

Long-standing anovulatory cycles produce endometrial changes that can be seen in an EB. As mentioned in Q. no. 15 (page 131), EB also serves as a test for ovulation and LPD.

Q6. When do you do endometrial biopsy in a menstrual cycle and why? What all tests are done on the biopsy specimen?

Endometrial biopsy is done in the premenstrual phase because during menstruation, the endometrium sheds off and neither the tubercular bacilli nor the histopathological changes can be detected at that time.

EB is an OPD procedure. The sampling is done with EB curette which does not require any cervical dilatation. In our hospital, we do EB in the minor (family planning) OT on OPD basis. The sample is taken from endometrial area near the tubal cornua (because tuberculosis spreads from fallopian tubes to the endometrium and the areas near cornua are initially involved). The sample is taken in 2 vials: one for AFB smear and culture (in a vial containing saline) and the other for histopathology (in a vial containing formalin).

4th visit 16.05.08

HSG report → B/L blocked tubes

Plan - Diagnostic hysteroscopy to evaluate uterine cavity and laparoscopy to confirm tubal block and tuboplasty at same sitting depending on site of block

Investigations for PAC

Follow up after diagnostic laparoscopy or tuboplasty

Counselling if tubes irreversibly blocked → IVF – ET/voluntary adoption

If no conception post 6 months of tuboplasty, repeat HSG → recurrence of tubal block → IVF-ET/voluntary adoption

Q7. If HSG is done in a case of genital tuberculosis, what findings will be suggestive?

As mentioned in the answer to Q4, HSG is not done in a suspected case of genital tuberculosis. However, if it is done in unsuspected case, the following findings can be seen:

1. Irregular filling of the uterine cavity if endometrial adhesions present, distorted contour of the cavity, vascular intravasation of the dye;
2. B/L tubal block in the isthmic region;
3. Beaded appearance of the tubes;
4. Rigid lead pipe appearance of the tubes;
5. Terminal Hydrosalpinx;
6. Tobacco pouch appearance of the fimbrial end; and
7. Peritubal adhesions leading to loculated spill of the dye.

CASE 10E UNEXPLAINED OR ENDOMETRIOSIS-RELATED INFERTILITY

2nd visit

Continued from **Case 10D**

HSA WNL

Follicular monitoring Ovulatory cycles

3rd visit

HSG B/L tubes patent

Plan Diagnostic laparoscopy to rule out peritoneal factors

PAC

Laparoscopy with dye test

Normal → Δ unexplained fertility I

OR

Peritoneal endometriotic implants with patent tubes → Burn the lesions with cautery or LASER. II

I. Δ Unexplained infertility

- Ovulation induction with intrauterine insemination (IUI) (3–4 cycles)
- If no conception → IVF-ET

II. Δ endometriosis

- Surgical therapy by laparoscopy followed by ovulation induction with IUI.
- If no conception in 3–6 cycles:
  - Refer for IVF-ET

Q1. When the diagnosis was established as endomteriosis, you advised surgery. Is there no role for medical treatment in endometriosis-related infertility?

Studies have shown that medical treatment is of no benefit for infertility associated with endometriosis.

Q2. One of the differential diagnosis is unexplained infertility. How is unexplained infertility defined? What are the management options for unexplained infertility?

When investigations of infertility fail to reveal a cause, i.e. semen is normal, ovulation is documented and tubes are patent with no peritoneal factor, this is labelled as unexplained infertility. This does not indicate the absence of a cause, but rather inability to identify it. The results of IVF have shown that there may be undiagnosed problems of oocyte or embryo quality or of implantation failure – none of which can be easily tested.

As exact cause is not known, the treatment is empirical. Expectant management, ovulation induction with-or-without IUI, and IVF-ET are the main approaches to treat it. One has to individualize treatment. Young couples or couples with secondary infertility might achieve pregnancy within 3 years of conservative or expectant treatment.

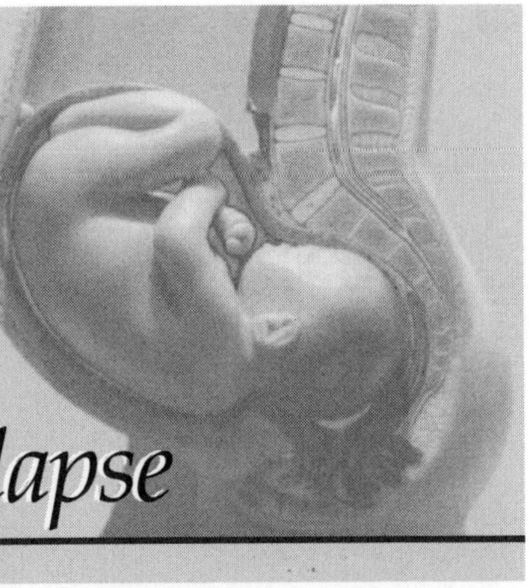

11 Uterovaginal Prolapse

Q1. You have asked the patient if she has associated urinary and anal incontinence. You have even examined the patient for SUI. Do these conditions tend to coexist with uterovaginal prolapse?

Yes, these conditions can coexist with uterovaginal prolapse and need to be taken care of during surgical repair.

Q2. You have diagnosed the case as stage-3 uterine prolapse. How is the staging done for a prolapse?

Earlier, prolapse was graded into 4 clinical stages subjectively as follows:

- *Stage I:* Descent of cervix or vaginal walls below the level of ischial spines or to the vaginal midplane
- *Stage II:* Descent to the hymenal ring
- *Stage III:* Descent to outside the introitus
- *Stage IV:* Complete eversion (procidentia), i.e. fundus of uterus can be felt outside the introitus.

Though used by many clinicians, the above-mentioned system has lot of inter-observer variations and the defects are not clear from this system. Therefore it is now recommended that prolapse should be staged according to POP-Q examination (pelvic organ prolapse quantification examination) proposed by

CASE 11A

XYZ 32-years F P_3 L_3, family completed, Not using any contraception

1st visit

C/o

Dragging sensation in the perineum
Something coming out of the introitus

HOPI

H/o chronic constipation
H/o of incomplete evacuation of bladder
No h/o bowel symptoms
No h/o chronic cough
No h/o urinary incontinence

Menstrual history:

4/30 days, regular, LMP- 10 days back

O/E

GPE – normal, average height and weight

Local examination:

- External genitalia normal
- No stress urinary incontinence
- On straining cervix comes out of introitus

- Decubitus ulcer present
- Cystocele outside the hymenal ring, rugae on vaginal wall absent, paravaginal sulci maintained.

No enterocele

Rectocele till the level of hymen

Perineal body 2 cm

P/V examination:

Prolapse is reducible. Uterus retroverted, normal size, mobile, supravaginal elongation of cervix present. Bilateral fornices are free. Levator tone poor (pap Smear to be taken before P/V examination)

- *POP- Q examination:* Aa +1, Ba +2, C +3, D -2, Ap +1, Bp +1, Pb 2, gh 5, tvl 10 cm
- Prolapse stage 3

Diagnosis:

32 year, P_3 L_3 with stage 3 uterine prolapse with cystocele +++, rectocele ++, no enterocele without SUI, with decubitus ulcer

Adv:

- Pap smear taken
- Glycerine acriflavin tampooning daily to reduce the prolapse
- Counsel the patient for surgery and tubal ligation
- Stool softeners
- Plan: Fothergill's operation with anterior colporrphy with posterior colpoperineorrhaphy with laparoscopic tubal ligation
- Investigations for PAC
- One unit blood donation for surgery

2nd visit

Get PAC , operate in postmenstrual period

international continence society (ICS), shown in Table 11.1. POP-Q ensures uniformity in nomenclature and objectively quantifies the prolapse.

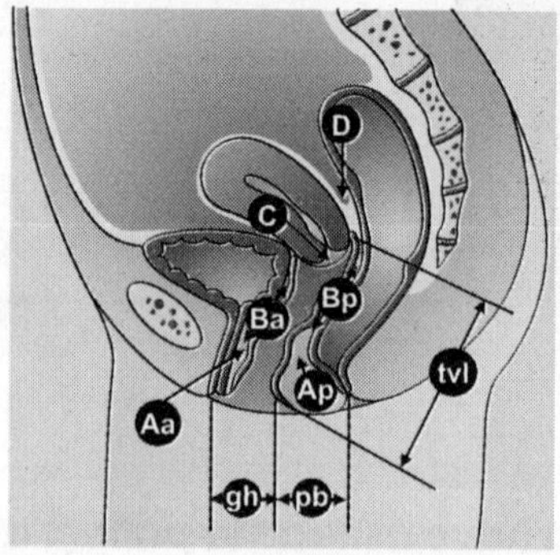

Source: Bump RC, Mattiasson A, Bo K, et al. The standardization of terminology of female pelvic organ prolapse and pelvic floor dysfunction. *Am J Obstet Gynecol.* 1996;175:13.

Fig. 11.1

There are 6 points measured at the vagina with respect to the hymen (Fig. 11.1).

- Points above the hymen are negative numbers; points below the hymen are positive numbers.

Point	*Description*	*Range of values*
Aa	Anterior vaginal wall 3 cm proximal to the hymen	–3 cm to + 3 cm
Ba	Most distal position of the remaining upper anterior vaginal wall	–3 cm to + tvl
C	Most distal edge of cervix or vaginal cuff scar	
D	Posterior fornix (N/A if post-hysterectomy)	
Ap	Posterior vaginal wall 3 cm proximal to the hymen	–3 cm to + 3 cm
Bp	Most distal positon of the remaining upper posterior vaginal wall	–3 cm to + tvl

Genital hiatus (gh)—Measured from middle of external urethral meatus to posterior midline hymen

Perineal body (pb)—Measured from posterior margin of gh to middle of anal opening

Total vaginal length (tvl)—Depth of vagina when point D or C is reduced to normal position

All measurements are taken from hymenal ring
Tvl is taken without straining.
Rest points are marked at full valsalva maneuver

Table 11.1: Staging based on POP-Q examination– ICS

Stage 0	No prolapse, Aa, Ap, Ba, Bp = –3 cm and C or D ≤ tvl–2 cm
Stage 1	Stage 0 criteria not met and leading edge of prolapse is <–1 cm
Stage 2	Most distal edge of prolapse ≥ –1 cm but ≤ +1 cm
Stage 3	Most distal edge > +1 cm but <+ (tvl–2) cm
Stage 4	Total eversion of genital tract, leading edge ≥ + (tvl–2) cm

Q3. Is the decubitus ulcer common in prolapse? What causes it?

Decubitus ulcer is commonly associated with third degree prolapse. Decubitus ulcers are ulcers on the cervix or prolapsed vaginal walls. These ulcers do not occur due to infection or mechanical friction. It is a trophic ulcer and occurs due to venous stasis there is less oxygenation of dependant tissues resulting in ulceration of vaginal mucosa. This needs to be healed by vaginal packing before surgical treatment.

Q4. How is decubitus ulcer treated?

The decubitus ulcer has to be completely healed before we take the patient for surgery.

- Keep the prolapse reduced with tampoon or pessary. Tampoon is soaked in glycerine acriflavin solution. Glycerine dehydrates the tissues and reduces edema while acriflavin is antiseptic.
- There is no need for antibiotics and it heals by one-to-two weeks
- If no healing–Rule out malignancy by Papanicolaou smear, colposcopy and directed biopsy if indicated. To promote healing one can use estrogens oral (tablet premarin 0.625 mg OD × 15 days) or vaginal oestradiol cream.

Q5. Why are the obstetric history, menstrual history important?

Obstetric history is important because prolapse is commoner in multiparous women. Moreover, it is important to know the future desire for fertility. It is important to elicit the menstrual history for acertaining if there is any associated menstrual problem that requires investigation before treatment. This may also have an implication on the treatment, e.g. if there is fibroid uterus causing menorrhagia, hysterectomy may be preferable to conservative surgery.

Q6. Why does the pap smear have to be taken before doing a P/V?

Pap smear is prepared from exfoliated cervical cells from transformation zone. P/V examination removes those cells and the smear prepared after P/V examination is likely to be inadequate.

Q7. How is prolapse treated?

Definitive treatment for prolapse surgery (Table 11.2).

Table 11.2: Broad choice of treatment

Pelvic floor exercise	1. Useful only for stage-I or II prolapse. 2. It will prevent the progress of prolapse but will not cure the existing descend.
Pessary	1. Effective for women who have significant medical problems and are poor risk for surgical treatment. 2. Pregnancy 3. While patient is waiting for surgery
Surgery	It is the mainstay of treatment. Surgery is tailored according to type of defect and reconstructive surgery is done, i.e. site of defect is identified and site specific defect is treated and adequate length of vagina is reconstructed.

Q8. What are the surgeries commonly done in our hospital for prolapse?

Vaginal hysterectomy with anterior colporrhaphy (if cystocele present) with McCall's Culdeplasty (if entrocele present) with posterior colpoperineorrhaphy (if rectocele, perineal defect present). Sacrospino colpopexy (Attaching the vaginal vault with sarospinous ligament) is also done with the procedure in cases of massive prolapse and procidentia.

Fothergill Manchester Repair in Multiparous women who desire to retain menstrual function.

Sling Surgeries in Nulliparous prolapse.

Sacral Colpopexy or Sacrospinous Colpopexy in Vault prolapse with anterior and posterior repair as required.

Q9. What are the main components of Fothergill's (Manchester) Operation?

This is a conservative surgery for prolapse. Main components are:

- Anterior colporrhaphy
- Amputation of cervix
- Cut ends of mackenrodt ligaments sutured in front of amputated cervix
- New cervical lips formed with vaginal mucosa
- Colpoperineorrhaphy.

Q10. Why have you decided for Manchester repair in the present case?

As she is a young woman, option of conservative surgery to retain menstrual function has been given.

Q11. So, in all young women presenting with prolapse we should do Fothergill's (Manchester) Operation?

No, this surgery is done when prolapse is due to obstetrical injury to the facial tissue while ligament support to the uterus is well maintained. This is not a suitable operation if ligaments are weak as in Nulliparous prolapse.

Q12. What is a Nulliparous prolapse and how do you manage that?

Nulliparous prolapse is a type of UV prolapse where the chief cause is inherent weakness of the Uterine support provided by the ligaments. This can occur at any age group with added injuries to the pelvic supports during child birth or further weakness after menopause, but most typically it presents in the young age group without any obstetrical cause.

Surgery done for Nulliparous prolapse in a young female is sling operation.

Abdominal sling operations are done in the cases of prolapse with following characteristics:

- Young women suffering from 2nd or 3rd degree prolapse
- Desirous of retaining childbearing and menstrual functions
- Nulliparous prolapse.

Objective

To buttress the weakened supports (Mackenrodt's and uterosacral ligamnets) of the uterus by providing a substitute as slings to support the uterus. Various Abdominal sling operations are:

- Abdominocervicopexy (Purandare's Sling operation)
  - Sling from rectus sheath attaching anterior isthmus to external oblique aponeurosis
- Shirodker's
  - Mersilene tape, attached to cervix posteriorly, retroperitoneally to anterior uterosacral ligament

Table 11.3: Differentiating features of uterine prolapse in young females requiring conservative surgery

	Nulliparous	*Multiparous*
Cause	Congenital weakness in Ligament support	Obsterical injury to the facial supports
Associated finding with uterine prolapse	Enterocele++ Cystocele, rectocele generally not there	Cystocele+++, Rectocele++
Cervical elongation	Absent	Present (Supravaginal)
Sugery	Sling Operation	Fothergill's Operation
Future pregnancy	Possible	Not advisable. Generally surgery done after lap ligation, as risk during future pregnancies are very high

- Khanna's
  - Mersilene tape, attached to posterior cervix at isthmus, thro broad ligament, attached to anterior superior iliac spine

Q13. So if a young woman comes with utero-vaginal prolapse, how do we differen-tiate between different conservative surgeries?

Differentiating features between two types of prolapses seen in young women are as shown in Table 11.3.

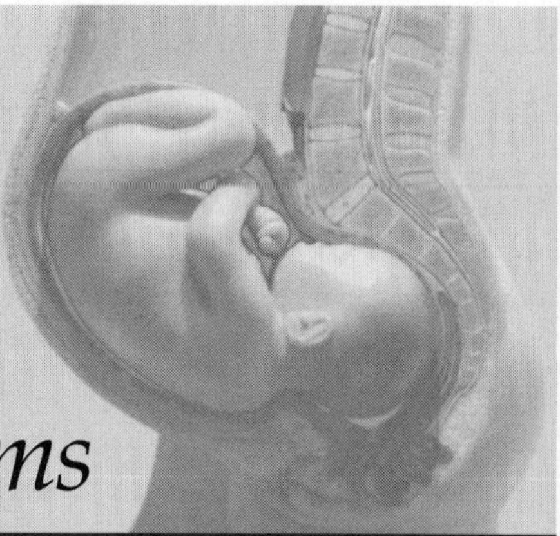

12 Urinary Symptoms

CASE 12A URGE INCONTINENCE DUE TO DETRUSOR OVERACTIVITY (DO)

ABC 40-years P_2

1st visit

C/o

Frequency urine – 3 months

Urge incontinence – 2 months

H/o

Nocturia +

No h/o hematuria/pain abdomen/fever

M/h: Normal cycles, LMP – 10 days back.

Past history

No h/o diabetes

O/E

General and systemic examination – NAD

P/A

No suprapubic or renal angle tenderness

P/S

No stress urinary incontinence

Cx and vagina healthy

Q1. You have recorded that the patient complains of 'urge' incontinence. Are there other types of urinary incontinence too?

Yes, urinary incontinence (leakage of urine) can be of different types (Table 12.1) that can usually be inferred by eliciting a detailed history.

Q2. Case 12A pertains to a patient having both urinary infection and detrusor overactivity. How often does urinary infection coexist with the different types of (urge, stress, continuous) incontinence?

Though the exact incidence is not known, urinary tract infections are more commonly seen in women with urinary incontinence and especially urge incontinence and less commonly with stress incontinence. Urinary infections are not the cause of continuous incontinence, but urinary fistulas are very often associated with UTI.

Q3. What would you do if, in a patient presenting with urge incontinence, the urine is sterile and the cystometrogram indicates a stable bladder (i.e. without detrusor overactivity)?

In that case, we shall refer the case to a urosurgeon or a urogynecologist. Further

Table 12.1: Definitions of various types of urinary incontinence

Urge urinary incontinence	Involuntary leakage accompanied by or immediately preceded by urgency. It is usually due *to urinary infection* or due to *detrusor overactivity/ instability* (DO). Less commonly, it is due to *genuine stress incontinence* (GSI).
Stress urinary incontinence (SUI)	Involuntary leakage of urine associated with an increase in intra-abdominal pressure, as during sneezing, coughing, laughing or running. It is usually due to *genuine stress incontinence* (GSI) but can be also due to *urinary infection* or due to *detrusor overactivity/ instability* (DO).
Continuous urinary incontinence	Continuous leakage of urine through the urethra indicates presence of overflow incontinence as in the neurogenic bladder. However, continuous leakage of urine per vaginum indicates a vesicovaginal fistula (VVF).

investigations would include an USG (to rule out bladder calculi or bladder growth), and cystoscopy or IVP to rule out interstitial cystitis.

Q4. You have prescribed tolterodine for the treatment of DO. What are the alternatives if tolterodine is not available?

Pharmacological treatment of detrusor overactivity involves administration of antimuscarinic agents, and tolterodine is only one of them. We can also prescribe *oxybutynin* 2.5 × tds × 3 months. Additionally, *imipramine* can be prescribed 75 mg HS for 3 months. Tolterodine is the first line drug, however in older patients imipramine can be the first option if depression seems associated symptom.

P/V
Uterus R/V, NS. fx free

Investigations:
1. Urine R & M E
2. Urine C/S
3. Blood sugar F & PP

Adv:
Review after investigation

2nd visit

Blood sugar	Normal
Urine M/E	Pus cells +ve > 5/HPF, No RBCs
Urine c/s	Shows growth

R_x
Tab. Norflox 400 mg BD × 3 days or antibiotic according to c/s report
Plenty of fluids
Repeat culture after antibiotics

3rd visit
Repeat culture sterile
Patient still symptomatic

Adv:
Frequency-volume charting for 72 hours
Cystometry to rule out detrusor overactivity

4th visit
Cystometry report indicates DO (detrusor overactivity) *see* Box 12.1

R_x
Tab tolterodine 2 mg BD × 3 months
Pelvic floor exercises
Bladder retraining and bladder drill

To report after 3 months for review.

Q5. Why do you test for urine R/M and C/S before treating UTI?

The treatment depends on the urine report (both R/m and C/s) which may show:

1. Positive urine culture (indicating bacterial infection) or
2. Sterile urine with pyuria (indicating absence of bacteria but presence of pus cells in urine).

Positive urine culture is treated with antibiotics to which the bacteria is most sensitive. This is indicated in the C/s report itself (Table 12.2 indicates the antibiotics of choice, just in case the sensitivity report is not available) For acute, uncomplicated cystitis, short-term (3 day course) therapy is preferable. Repeat negative culture after completion of therapy indicates cure. The treatment includes:

1. Antibiotic × 3 days (usually Norfloxacin 400 mg BD × 3 days)
2. Plenty of oral fluids × 3 days
3. Alkacitron (sodium citrate solution 2 tsf BD × 3 days)

Recurrent urinary tract infection may occur due to relapse of original or to reinfection with the same or a different organism. These patients are advised:

1. Blood sugar (fasting and PP) to rule out diabetes mellitus,
2. Ultrasound KUB (to rule out calculi), and
3. Estrogen vaginal cream in postmenopausal.

If no cause found, the patient should be referred to the urogynecologist for further investigations.

Sterile urine culture with pyuria on microscopy may suggests chlamydial infection or tuberculosis. Suspect chlamydial infection if history is short. Laboratory tests for Chlamydia are expensive and not easily available. It is treated with either Tab Azithromyin 1 g orally in a single dose, or cap doxycycline (100 mg) 1 BD × 7 days. Urinary tuberculosis is suspected if symptoms are for long duration with sterile pyuria. Get urinary AFB smear staining and culture in 24 hours urinary sample. Positivity of AFB in urine demands evaluation of upper urinary tract, i.e. kidneys and kidney function tests.

Table 12.2: Antibiotic treatment for UTI

Bacteria	*Antibiotic prescribed*
Gram-negative bacilli (Examples: *E. coli, Klebsiella*)	Norfloxacin Ciprofloxacin Gentamycin
Gram-positive bacilli (*Staphylococcus,* *Streptococcus*)	Sulphonamide Cotrimoxazole Trimethoprim Nitrofurantoin
Pseudomonas	Norfloxacin Ciprofloxacin Gentamycin

Q6. How will you treat a patient with urgency, nocturia and dysuria if the urine is sterile and without pyuria?

Sterile urine culture without pyuria, when associated with lower urinary tract (LUT) symptoms (frequency, urgency, nocturia, dysuria) in combination with pain is called "painful bladder syndrome" which has varied etiology and is a difficult group to treat.

1. Get 72 hours urinary diary (*see* Annexure 12.1)
2. Urinary cytology
3. Cystometry (urodynamic study) to rule out detrusor instability
4. Cystoscopy and treatment accordingly.

Q1. What is genuine stress incontinence and how is it different from stress Incontinence?

Stress urinary incontinence (SUI) is a symptom while genuine stress incontinence (GSI) is a condition. GSI is the commonest cause of SUI but it can also cause the symptom of urge incontinence. Similarly, urinary infection and detrusor overactivity are common causes of urge incontinence but they occasionally give rise to the symptom of SUI. Hence, in both SUI and urge incontinence, it is important to rule out urinary infection (through urine C/s) and detrusor overactivity (through cystometry, *see* Box 12.1) before arriving at the diagnosis of GSI.

Q2. You have advised pelvic floor exercises. What are other non-surgical modalities for GSI?

It is the usual practice to first offer conservative management comprising:

1. Pelvic floor exercises,

Box 12.1: Cystometry

In the normal bladder, the first sensation of bladder filling occurs when about 150 ml fluid has been infused, and a strong desire to void occurs at about 450 ml and has normal compliance, i.e. no associated tonic rise in bladder pressure on filling.

Detrusor over activity (DO) or instability is diagnosed when involuntary detrusor contraction occurs during the filling phase of cystometry, which may be spontaneous or provoked (e.g. provoked by cough, washing hands in cold water, sound of running water).

Genuine stress incontinence (GSI) is diagnosed if leakage of urine occurs on coughing in the absence of a rise in detrusor pressure.

CASE 12B STRESS INCONTINENCE DUE TO GENUINE STRESS INCONTINENCE (GSI)

DEF 40 years P_2 female

1st visit

C/o

Stress urinary incontinence – 6 months

No h/o urge incontinence/frequency of urine/ nocturia

No h/o uterovaginal prolapse

M/h

Normal cycles, LMP 10 days back

O/E

General systemic examination–normal

P/A NAD

Local examination:

Examination with full bladder: SUI (Stress urinary incontinence) + No latent period between coughing and urinary leak.

P/S: No cervical descent

No cystocele or rectocele

P/V: Ut R/V, NS, fx free

Δ SUI

Investigations:

Urine C/s

2nd visit

Urine sterile

Adv: Cystometry

3rd visit

Cystometry: GSI

Δ GSI

*R*x
Counselling for modalities of treatment
Pelvic exercises with vaginal cones in Physiotherapy Department × 3 months followed by reevaluation

3rd visit
No improvement

Adv:
TVT-O sling (Transvaginal tape–obturator sling)
Investigate for PAC

2. Vaginal cones or weights. This consists of set of preweighted cones which patient tries to hold in vagina. By doing this she contracts her pelvic muscles and gradually vaginal cones of increasing weight are used. This provides biofeedback to the patient. Electrostimulation and mechanical devices are employed when the exercises and cones fail.
3. In electrostimulation, current is applied to pelvic muscles using perineal or vaginal electrodes. Patient feels the pelvic muscles contract, providing biofeedback to the patient for performing the pelvic exercises better.
4. Intravaginal mechanical devices (e.g. contiform device) elevates the bladder neck while urethral mechanical devices plug the urethra to prevent leakage.

Q3. In the third visit, you advised TVT-O to the patient. What is TVT-O? Why did you advice PAC to the patient?

PAC was advised because the patient needed surgery. Surgical treatment usually takes the form of:

1. Midurethral sling with transobturator tension free tape (TVT-O) using the vaginal approach.
2. Burch's suspension (using the abdominal approach).

The choice of conservative management versus surgical approach must take into consideration the patient's QOL (quality of life) and *her* choice of treatment.

Q1. What are the causes of VVF and what is the cause in this case?

Common causes of VVF are listed in Box 12.2. The present case is of obstetric fistula which resulted because of ischaemic necrosis as there is history of prolonged labour and onset of urinary leak is after 7 days.

Q2. From Box 12.2 (common causes of VVF), it is clear that the obstetric history is important in etiology of continuous incontinence. Is it also important in other types of incontinence?

Yes, obstetric injury (difficult delivery, delivery of a big baby) may also be responsible for stress incontinence. Multiple vaginal births result in cystocele causing anatomical descent of bladder neck and loss of its sphicteric control during increased intra-abdominal pressure.

Q3. How do you manage VVF?

The management of VVF involves the following steps: First, the history of the illness

Box 12.2: Common causes of vesicovaginal fistulae

- After prolonged and difficult delivery (*obstetric fistula*)
  - Due to trauma of instrumental delivery (leakage starts immediately after delivery)
  - Due to ischemia and pressure necrosis of anterior vaginal wall and posterior bladder wall as this gets impacted between the fetal head and pubic symphysis (leakage starts about 7 days after delivery)
- After caesarean section or gynecological surgery – operative trauma
- After radiation therapy
- Due to malignancy or tuberculosis, and rarely, schistosomiasis.

CASE 12C CONTINUOUS INCONTINENCE (VESICO-VAGINAL FISTULA)

22 years $P_{1+0+0+0}$

C/o
Continuous dribbling of urine – 6 months

H/o
Prolonged labour followed by caesarian section 6 months back. Dribbling of urine started 7 days after the operation. She had catheter in situ for 14 days postoperative period. She was discharged after removal of catheter.

O/H
$P_{1+0+0+0}$. It was a stillborn baby with hydrocephalus, delivered by cesarean section after 2 days of labour pains at home

M/H
Patient is amenorrheic.

O/E
Short statured 4'' height
Smells of urine
General systemic examination – NAD

Local examination – vulvar excoriations ++

P/s
Big (1 × 1 cm) hole in the anterior mid-vagina, bladder mucosa protruding through hole. Urine coming through it.

P/V
Single fistula with fibrosis all around it. Not fixed to the pubic bone.
Cx ↓, Ut A/V NS, fx free
Δ Vesicovaginal fistula

Investigations
Urine C/s and investigations for PAC
Admit to ward for 3-swab test, evaluation of fistula, cystoscopy and repair by flap-splitting method.

is elicited to find out how the leakage started. Next, the anterior vaginal wall is examined after retracing posterior vaginal wall with Sim's speculum to look for the number, site and size of fistulous openings. Per vaginum examination is done to note the fibrosis around fistulous margin and fixity of fistula to pubic bone. Such fistulae are difficult to repair and one might have to use graft or modified technique and have to be handled by experienced surgeons. The three swab test (*B*ox 12.3) is performed. The test differentiates between ureteric and vesical fistulae and management of ureteric fistulae is altogether different from vesical fistulae. Thereafter, an urine sample is collected in Sim's speculum for urine culture. Cystoscopy is performed to know the number, site and size of fistula and its relationship to ureteric openings. Vulvar excoriations are treated with vaseline or ZnO cream, and the PAC is performed.

Surgery for VVF repair (e.g. by Flap splitting method) is planned atleast 3 months after the initial insult. This gives time to the tissues to recover from local congestion and edema. Sometimes the fistula decreases in size due to fibrosis.

Q4. What are principles of VVF repair?

Principles for VVF repair are:

1. Urine culture should be sterile
2. Good exposure and good light–90% fistulae can be approached by per vaginum route
3. Microinstruments and fine sutures (2–0 or 3–0 Vicryl)
4. Hemostasis
5. Good mobilization of bladder mucosa from vagina
6. No tension in sutures
7. Postoperative continuous drainage of bladder–dual drainage is better, i.e. Suprapubic cystostomy and per urethral Foley's catheter drainage for 14 days.

Q5. Can the woman lead a normal life after fistula repair?

Yes, but at the time of discharge, she is advised abstinence for 3 months and to ensure that the next delivery is by caesarean section.

Box 12.3: The 3-swab test

1. Catheterize bladder
2. Put three cotton swabs in vagina
   - No-1 At the vaginal vault
   - No-2 In the midvagina
   - No-3 At the introitus
3. Instill 100-200 cc of 1% methylene blue in bladder through catheter
4. Remove the swab after 5–10 minutes.

Swab 3

- Blue staining–discard it as this may be due to overflow from catheter

Swab 2

- Blue staining–vesicovaginal fistula (VVF)
- Dry swab – No VVF

Swab 1

- Dry – No ureteric fistula
- Wet but not stained blue – ureteric fistula

Annexure 12.1

Frequency-volume chart (urinary diary)

Day 1			Day 2			Day 3		
Time	*Volume (ml)*	*Episodes of urge incontinence*	*Time*	*Volume (ml)*	*Episodes of urge incontinence*	*Time*	*Volume (ml)*	*Episodes of urge incontinence*
6:00 am			6:00 am			6:00 am		
7:00 am			7:00 am			7:00 am		
8:00 am			8:00 am			8:00 am		
9:00 am			9:00 am			9:00 am		
10:00 am			10:00 am			10:00 am		
11:00 am			11:00 am			11:00 am		
12:00 pm			12:00 pm			12:00 pm		
1:00 pm			1:00 pm			1:00 pm		
2:00 pm			2:00 pm			2:00 pm		
3:00 pm			3:00 pm			3:00 pm		
4:00 pm			4:00 pm			4:00 pm		
5:00 pm			5:00 pm			5:00 pm		
6:00 pm			6:00 pm			6:00 pm		
7:00 pm			7:00 pm			7:00 pm		
8:00 pm			8:00 pm			8:00 pm		
9:00 pm			9:00 pm			9:00 pm		
10:00 pm			10:00 pm			10:00 pm		
11:00 pm			11:00 pm			11:00 pm		
12:00 am			12:00 am			12:00 am		
1:00 am			1:00 am			1:00 am		
2:00 am			2:00 am			2:00 am		
3:00 am			3:00 am			3:00 am		
4:00 am			4:00 am			4:00 am		
5:00 am			5:00 am			5:00 am		

Information to be gathered from the chart:

(1) Total urinary output per day, (2) No. of voids per day, (3) Average volume of urine voided per day, (4) Nocturia (5) Episodes of urge incontinence

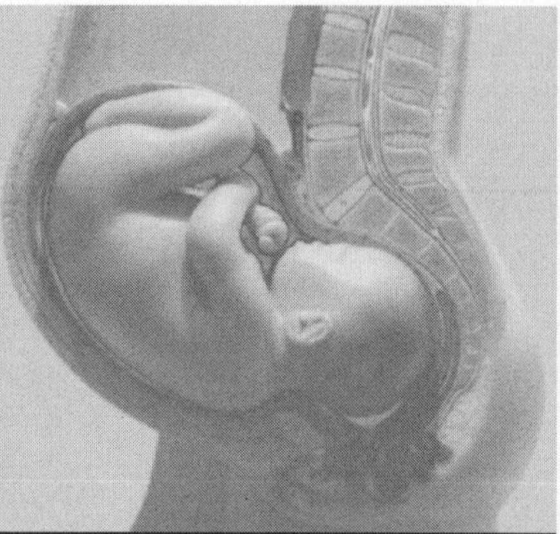

13 *Lump Abdomen*

CASE 13A LUMP ABDOMEN (OVARIAN CYST)

A 24-year-old Female, P_2 L_2

C/o

Heaviness and feeling of lump in lower abdomen 4 months

Mass is felt below umbilicus and is slowly increasing in size

No h/o pain, fever, anorexia, or loss of weight

No urinary or bowel complaints

LMP 10 days back

Normal menstrual cycles

O/E

General physical examination: NAD, no lymphadenopathy or pedal edema

Breast - Nad

P/A

Midline suprapubic cystic mass of 16 weeks gravid uterus size felt arising from pelvis which is more towards right side of abdomen

No free fluid in abdomen

Q1. Is not the patient too young to have an ovarian cyst?

No, ovarian cysts are quite common in all ages, affecting both premenopausal and postmenopausal woman. They can be functional (i.e. not pathological), neoplastic (benign or malignant) or endometrioma.

Q2. Why does P/A examination reveal a midline mass although it is a tumor of the right ovary?

Ovarian tumour has a pedicle because of which even one sided tumour can occupy midline position. However, on P/V examination this lump is felt through posterior fornix and is more towards right side.

Q3. You have recorded that the tumour is 'felt through right and posterior fornix'. What is the significance of this observation? If tumour is felt through anterior fornix, does it make any difference?

In case of lump which is felt through anterior fornix, one has to keep in mind, after ruling out full bladder, the strong possibility of parovarian cyst and dermoid ovarian cyst.

Q4. P/V examination reveals the cervix to be downward and forwards. Why is it important to mention it?

It is important to mention it because lateral tumours often push the cervix to one side.

Q5. You have mentioned "no nodularity in pouch of Douglas, rectal mucosa free". What is the significance of these observations?

In case of suspicion of ovarian neoplasm, the aim is to look for signs of malignancy. Nodularity is suggestive of secondaries and the 'free' rectal mucosa suggests the absence of any rectal involvement.

Q6. You have asked for an investigation on CA-125. What is CA-125?

Cancer antigen-125 (CA-125), is a protein that is present normally on cell membrane and is released in the bloodstream. It is present in higher concentration in most ovarian cancer cells, and in a postmenopausal woman with an ovarian tumor, a very high CA-125 level is highly suggestive of malignancy. However, the specificity of the test is low because CA-125 levels can be elevated in common benign conditions like endometriosis, PID, etc.

Q7. Suppose a patient presents with a similar lump in an abdomen which is NOT an ovarian cyst. At what stage would you refer her to the general surgeon–after clinical examination, after obtaining USG report, or after the report of CA-125?

If we are sure clinically that this tumour is not of gynecological (adenexal or uterine) origin, we can refer the patient to the surgery department. Else, we can take help of USG and other imaging methods to look for any adnexal or uterine pathology before referring the patient. Many a times, in cases of uncharacteristic tumor, the dilemma still

No hepato or splenomegaly

P/S Cervix and vagina healthy

P/v
Cervix anterior, deviated to left side
Uterus R/V, NS. mobile
Mobile, cystic mass, 12 × 12 cm, felt through right and posterior fornix, separate from uterus
Left fx - no mass,

P/V/R
No nodularity in pouch of douglas
Rectal mucosa free

CI
Rt. adnexal mass (? ovarian neoplasm)

Investigations:
USG – transabdominal and TVS

Next visit
USG – uterus and left ovary normal. On right side 12 × 12 cm, unilocular cyst seen with no sepatations and no solid areas. Rt ovary not seen
No free fluid in abdomen, liver echotexture normal

Diagnosis:
Right ovarian cyst

Adv:
Plan: Ovarian cystectomy/oophorectomy by laparoscopy

CA 125
Investigations for PACs

remains and is solved only at the time of exploratory laparotomy.

Q8. Can an ovarian cyst be mistaken for anything else?

Yes, the lumps that are commonly encountered and can be mistaken for an ovarian cyst are a full bladder, subserosal or broad ligament fibroid, hydrosalpinx, tubo-ovarian mass, A full bladder is ruled by history and examination, in case of doubt, simple catheterisation will resolve the controversy. Hydrosalpinx feels like a retort-shaped swelling with restricted mobility in posterior fornix and on USG, the ovaries are seen as separate from the mass. In case of a pelvic lump, one must look for both the kidneys on USG to confirm their normal location and rule out hydronephrosis which can result form pressure effects. If dilemma still exists, CAT scan/MRI would be prudent, but it has to be tailored according to the clinical situation.

Q9. How will you make out whether this tumour is benign or malignant?

The age and history and constitutional symptoms of the patient are suggestive. Ovarian masses are more likely to be malignant in postmenopausal age group and premenarchal girls as compared to reproductive age females. On examination, a solid, irregular, fixed pelvic mass, the presence of ascitis, bilaterality of tumour, evidence of secondaries are highly suggestive of malignancy. An USG can identify a normal ovary and thereby rule out malignancy with a high level of certainty. It can also detect certain features of malignancy in the ovarian cyst (e.g. thickened walls, irregular borders, solid areas, etc.) as well as some of the associated effects of malignancy such as hydronephrosis, ascites, and pleural effusions. However, since many physiological cysts and benign tumors have similar characteristics to malignancy, the specificity of ultrasound for ovarian cancer is low.

Q10. If this tumour seems benign, why do we need to remove it?

Preoperatively it is difficult to rule out malignancy with high accuracy. If not removed, it will grow and result in complications like torsion, haemorrhage in cyst, infection, rupture of cyst or malignant transformation. Premenopausal women with asymptomatic simple cysts smaller than 8 cm on sonograms and with normal CA125 value level may be monitored with a repeat ultrasonographic examination in 8–12 weeks. Hormone therapy, including the use of the oral contraceptive pill, is not helpful in causing resolution.

Q11. Is it safe to remove the ovarian cyst (cystectomy or oophrectomy) by laparoscopy?

Yes, provided one is confident of benign nature of the cyst. Since this case is of simple monolocular cyst with normal CA125 and RMI of less than 200, one can opt for laparoscopic removal. During laparoscopy, a thorough inspection is done first. If there is ascitis, the aspirate is sent for cytology, and a laparotomy is done if the cytology suggest any possibility of malignancy.

Q12. You seem to rely on the RMI for making a clinical decision. What is RMI?

RMI (risk of malignancy index) is an empirical index of malignancy derived from certain 'scores' alloted to the results of transvaginal ultrasound examination (U), menopausal status (M), and blood level (in U/ml) of the ovarian cancer marker CA125. It is given by the formula:

$$RMI = U \times M \times CA125.$$

A value of 200 or higher is taken as suggestive of malignancy.

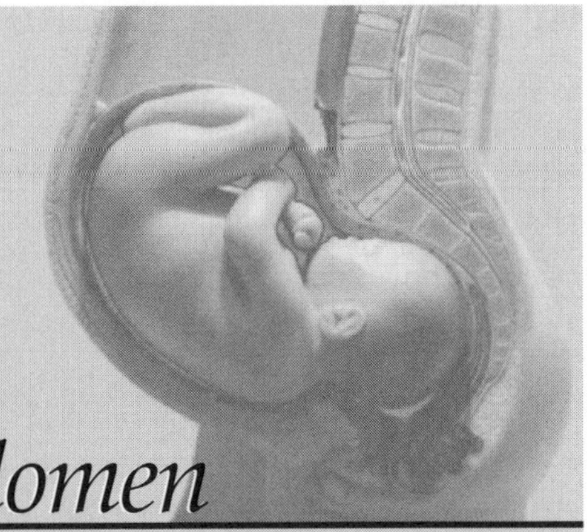

14 Acute Pain Abdomen

CASE 14A ACUTE PID

A 19-year-old female, P_1L_1

C/o
Acute lower abdominal pain
Fever for one day
Nausea and vomiting

Pain is severe, diffuse in lower abdomen with no h/o shifting or radiation of pain.
No aggravating or relieving factors.
No urinary or bowel complaints

LMP 10 days back
Had heavy bleeding this cycle
Previous cycles normal
P_1L_1, LCB 1 yr back, no contraception used

O/E
Febrile
Pulse 100/min
BP 120/80 mmHg

P/A
Generalized tenderness in lower abdomen
No mass/organomegaly/free fluid

Q1. What are the possibilities you consider when a patient comes with acute abdominal pain?

In a patient presenting with acute abdominal pain, we consider the gynaecological conditions that are *not* associated with hemoperitoneum (like acute PID and twisted ovarian cyst) and those that are associated with hemperitoneum (ruptured ectopic, perforating mole and corpus luteum hemorrhage). Non gynaecological causes like appendicitis, ureteric colic, etc are also to be ruled out.

Q2. Why did you ask about shifting pain? What would it indicate when present?

To rule out appendicitis. Pain of appendicitis starts in the umbilical area and shifts to right iliac fossa.

Q3. Does the heavy bleeding in the latest cycle signify anything in particular?

Patients of acute PID may have excessive menstrual bleeding due to endometritis.

Q4. You have recorded that there is 'no mass/organomegaly'. Why is it important to record it?

A mass felt per abdomen could be due to a huge tubo-ovarian (TO) abscess, twisted

Local
No pus from urethra
P/s
Cervix congested
Unhealthy discharge from os

P/v
Cervical excitation pain +
Uterus R/v, NS
Uterine movements tender
Rt TO mass 7 × 7 cm, very tender
Left fx no mass, but tenderness ++

P/v/R
No bulge in pouch of douglas

CI
Ac PID
Ectopic pregnancy to be ruled out

Adv:
Admit and investigate
Hemogram with ESR
Urine pregnancy test
Endocervical and high vaginal swab c/s
Urine (R and M/E)
Start I-V antibiotics
IV Cefoxitin 2 g 4 times daily +
IV Doxycycline 100 mg bd or oral Doxycycline if patient can tolerate

Watch for:
- Temp, pulse and respiratory rate 4 hourly
- Pain abdomen
- S/s peritonitis

Reports:
UPT – ve
Hb 10 g%

ovarian cyst or an appendicular lump. Organomegaly has to be noticed which can be part of multisystem pathology.

Q5. You have recorded, on local examination, that there is 'no pus from urethra'. Why is it important to record it?

Pus from the urethra indicates gonococcal urethritis. The pus should be subjected to Gram staining for Neisseria Gonococcus. It should be treated accordingly.

Q6. You have recorded, on P/s examination, that there is 'unhealthy discharge from os'. Does discharge from the os indicate pyometra?

Discharge from os could be due to endocervicitis or endometritis. Pyometra is diagnosed when there is associated enlarged uterus and USG shows collection of fluid in the uterus.

Q7. You have recorded, on P/V/R examination, that there is 'no bulge' in the pouch of Douglas. Why?

A bulge in POD signifies collection in pelvis, pelvic abscess or pelvic hematocoel.

Q8. Did you have anything specific in mind when you advised ESR estimation?

To differentiate PID from ectopic pregnancy in acute pain abdomen: Raised ESR in presence of normal Hb and increased TLC indicates ac PID, however raised ESR with normal Hb and TLC might indicate chronic infection, i.e. tuberculosis.

Q9. How do you define pelvic inflammatory disorder and briefly mention its causes?

PID is defined as an ascending infection of the female upper genital tract (structures above the cervix). It is mostly caused by STDs but also occurs following postpartum, postabortal (either miscarriage or abortion) or intrauterine device (IUD) related infections. The etiology of PID is polymicrobial. Sexually transmitted infections are mostly caused by *Chlamydia* and *N.gonorrhoeae*. Other causative organisms include anaerobes causing bacterial vaginosis, enteric gram-negative rods and streptococci.

PID is more likely to occur when there is a history of an earlier episode of the same, recent sexual contact with a partner with STD, recent onset of menses (PID occurs mostly in postmensrual phase because blood is good culture medium for bacteria), or if an IUD is in place.

Q10. What is the differential diagnosis of PID? Is ectopic pregnancy one of its causes, or is it important in differential diagnosis?

The differential diagnosis of PID includes appendicitis, ectopic pregnancy, septic abortion, hemorrhagic or ruptured ovarian cysts or tumors, twisted ovarian cyst, degeneration of a myoma, and acute enteritis. The first step in narrowing down the differential diagnosis is to do a urinary pregnancy test.

If the urine pregnancy test is positive, ectopic pregnancy remains a possibility. If the ectopic pregnancy is of over six weeks, it can be confirmed using pelvic and vaginal ultrasounds. If USG is not conclusive and their is fluid in the pelvis, **culdocentesis** should be done to differentiate hemoperitoneum (ruptured ectopic pregnancy or hemorrhagic cyst) from pelvic sepsis (salpingitis, ruptured pelvic abscess, or ruptured appendix).

If the urine pregnancy test is negative, it must be reconfirmed with the more sensitive serum pregnancy test to rule out ectopic pregnancy depending on the clinical degree of suspicion. Laparoscopy is often done to diagnose pelvic inflammatory disease, and it is imperative if the diagnosis is not certain or if the patient has not responded to antibiotic therapy after 48 hours.

TLC 14,000/cc
ESR 40 mm 1st hour

Pelvic USG

Uterus normal, ET 10 mm, Right adenexal heterogenous mass with absent fire sign on color Doppler, minimal fluid present around uterus

Endocervical and high vaginal swab c/s – no growth

Urine (R and M/E)–normal, no pus cells

Review after 24 hours

Patient improving

Continue I-V A/B for 24 hours more

Review after 24 hours

Switch over to oral antibiotics:

Oral doxycycline 100 mg twice daily plus oral metronidazole 400 mg twice daily for total of 14 days.

Patient stable

To be discharged with advice of abstinence till recovery and partner's workup in genitor urinary medicine clinic.

Q11. What is culdocentesis? What do we look for while doing culdocentesis?

Culdocentesis is needle aspiration of cul-de-sac. Whenever there is collection in POD, culdocentesis tells us nature of collected fluid, e.g., it may be pus (in pelvic abscess) or blood (in pelvic haematocele or hemoperitoneum).

Q12. Do you stop antibiotic therapy if the culture report is not positive?

The culture report may not be positive in all the cases because vaginal and endocervical secretions may not show the organisms at the time of endometrial or tubo-ovarian or pelvic peritoneal inflammation. Moreover, routine cultures do not test for Chlamydia. Hence, in case of clinical improvement one should continue the antibiotics even if cultures are negative.

Q13. What are the alternative antibiotic regimens for treatment of PID? How do they compare with the cefoxitin/doxycycline regimen?

Etiological agents found in PID include *N. gonorrhoeae, C. trachomatis*, anaerobic bacteria, Gram-negative facultative bacteria, and streptococci. As it is impossible to differentiate between these clinically and a precise microbiological diagnosis is difficult, the treatment regimens must be effective against this broad range of pathogens. Partners of patients with PID should also be treated for gonorrhoea and chlamydia.

An alternative regimen is:

- Inj clindamycin IV 900 mg three times daily + Inj gentamicin IV 2 mg/kg loading dose followed by 1.5 mg/kg tds followed by
- Tab clindamycin 450 mg qid or cap doxycyline bid for 14 days + tab metronidazole 400 mg bid for 14 days

If the above regimens are not available, we give 14 days therapy to cover *N.gonorrhoeae* (quinolones, cephalosporins, penicillin) and *C. trachomatis* (tetracyclines, macrolides) and anaerobic bacteria (metronidazole).

Q14. What are indications of surgical intervention?

Surgical intervention is indicated in patients who have a questionable diagnosis or fail to respond to medical treatment within 72 hours or if there is a suspected rupture of TO abscess resulting in generalized peritonitis. Pelvic abscess is drained by colpotomy.

Q15. Does the patient always need to be hospitalized? If not, what outpatient treatment do you give to the patient?

Admission is necessary if the patient is severely ill and needs intravenous antibiotics. It is also necessary if she is an adolescent, is pregnant or has HIV, or if abdominal emergencies such as appendicitis cannot be ruled out. Other indications are if pelvic abscess is there . If during outdoor treatment the patient is unable to follow or tolerate an outpatient regimen; or the patient has failed to respond to outpatient therapy, she should be hospitalized.

If hospitalization is not necessary, antibiotics are prescribed immediately, since delaying treatment is risky. In addition to the drug treatment, bedrest and plenty of liquids are recommended. Sexual intercourse should be avoided until recovery is complete (often for two to three months). CDC recommends the following antibiotic treatments:

- Inj ceftriaxone 250 mg IM stat (for gonorrhoea) or
- Inj cefoxitin 2 g IM and tab probenecid 1 gm or
- Cefixime 400 mg single oral dose or
- Ciprofloxacin 500 mg single oral dose followed by:
- Cap doxycycline 100 mg bd (for Chlamydia) or tab ofloxacin 400 mg bd × 14 days + tab metronidazole (for anaerobes) 400 mg bid × 14 days

Q16. What are the likely complications if the PID is left untreated?

If untreated, PID may lead to serious complications, including life-threatening pelvic abscess, rupture of TO abscess, peritonitis and septicemia. Long-term complications of PID include ectopic pregnancies, infertility, and chronic pelvic pain.

Q17. How will you treat PID when you are not sure about its cause?

In such cases, we use the syndromic approach which is given without complete examination and tests. Paraprofessionals can use this approach. This concept was introduced by WHO. It is mostly with oral drugs and is based on the symptom complex. For syndrome of PID syndromic T/t is same as described above where we are giving treatment for all the causative organisms for PID (gonorrhoea, chlamydia and anerobes).

CASE 14B RUPTURED ECTOPIC PREGNANCY

A 30-year-old nulliparous woman with 6 weeks amenorrhoea
c/o severe pain abdomen for 3–4 hours associated with vomitings
H/o spotting P/V since yesterday
c/o fainting attacks since morning,
UPT +ve 1 week back
No USG done

Past history:
Married for 6 years. c/o primary infertility
Underwent tuboplasty for tubal block 1 year back
No h/o tuberculosis

O/E
Patient drowsy
pallor +++
Pulse: 120 min, low volume
BP: 80 mmHg systolic
RR: 30/min
Chest,CVS: NAD

P/A
Abdomen distended
Tenderness ++
Guarding +
Free fluid +

P/V
Cervix soft, cervical motion tenderness++
Fullness + in all fornices, tenderness ++
No mass palpable

Management:
Immediate resuscitation
Two I/V lines, give fast fluids (RL/DNS/NS)

Q1. Why do you say it is a case of ruptured ectopic?

As the patient is in the reproductive age group with positive urine pregnancy test, she is in early pregnancy. As clinically she is in hemorrhagic shock with hemoperitoneum, the first differential diagnosis is ruptured ectopic pegnancy. With USG showing absence of gestational sac in the uterus and a mixed echogenic mass in the adenexa confirms ectopic pregnancy.

Q2. Is past history significant in this case?

Yes, the history of infertility and tubal surgery makes the woman high risk for ectopic pregnancy.

Q3. What are other factors that make a woman high risk for ectopic pregnancy?

History of previous ectopic pregnancy, PID, genital TB, infertility, tubal surgery (tuboplasty, tubal recanalization), infertility treatment, tubal ligation, using CuT make a woman high risk case for ectopic pregnancy.

Q4. Do you mean that CuT increases the incidence of ectopic pregnancy?

No, CuT prevents all pregnancies including ectopic pregnancy as it is a very effective contraceptive method. Therefore with the use of CuT, the incidence of ectopic pregnancy decreases, but if pregnancy does occur with a CuT *in situ*, there is a greater chance that the pregnancy will be ectopic.

Q5. How will the knowledge of these high risk factors help in the management of patients?

It is important to be aware of these high risk factors so that if a woman with these factors conceives, one should keep a high suspicion of ectopic pregnancy and do early USG so as to detect ectopic pregnancy in unruptured state if possible. Detection in the unruptured state avoids mortality/morbidity associated with acute presentation (as in this case) and also allows the option of medical management thus avoiding surgery and also salvaging the uterine tube.

Q6. How would you arrive at a diagnosis if a USG is not available?

USG is not an absolute necessity in such an acute presentation. The management (surgery) should not be delayed for the USG. As the clinical diagnosis is almost certain and there is evidence of fluid in the abdomen, we can confirm hemoperitoneum by doing **paracentesis** (aspiration fluid trans-abdominally). Early pregnancy with hemoperitoneum almost always occurs due to ectopic pregnancy. Even otherwise, such a case will require urgent laparotomy to control source of hemorrhage, and therefore, the management remains the same.

Q7. Can we rule out hemoperitoneum if we do not get blood on paracentesis?

No. in massive hemoperitoeum (as evidenced clinically), paracentesis is confirmatory. However, in cases of lesser hemoperitoneum (as in cases of subacute presentation), blood mainly collects in the pelvic peritoneal cavity, which can be detected through a different procedure called 'culdocentesis'. Culdocentesis is aspiration of the blood from the cul-de-sac of peritoneal cavity through posterior vaginal fornix. The patient is put in lithotomy position, the posterior vaginal wall is retracted with the speculum, the posterior lip of cervix is held with volsellum to expose the posterior vaginal fornix. A sterile long intracath needle is inserted through posterior fornix to aspirate fluid from the cul-de-sac. If the aspirated blood does not clot, it confirms the presence of hemoperitoneum.

Arrange for cross-matched blood and transfuse as early as possible.
Oxygen by mask

Investigations:
Hb, platelet count, coagulation profile
UPT (if not already done)
Urgent USG (if available) for location of gestational sac, adenexal mass, free fluid

USG Report: Fluid present in abdomen
Uterine cavity empty
Mixed echogenic mass in right adenexa

Clinical diagnosis: Ruptured ectopic pregnancy
prepare for urgent laparotomy and salpingectomy

Q8. How long after the patient is resuscitated should the laparotomy be performed?

We should start resuscitation immediately and simultaneously make arrangements for laparotomy. The laparotomy (to control bleeding) should be done as soon as possible.

Q9. Are there any differential diagnoses in this case?

Other obstetric causes of spontaneous hemoperitoneum in early pregnancy can be corpus luteum hemorrhage and perforating molar pregnancy. One must always ask for history of any MTP or evacuation because perforation of uterus is common during these procedures. Even in these two cases, an urgent laparotomy is required to control bleeding.

CASE 14C TWISTED OVARIAN CYST

A 19-year-old female
C/o
Acute pain abdomen × 6 hours
Associated with vomitings
No h/o fever, urinary or bowel complaints
No h/o amenorrhea

Married for 6 months, nulliparous
Menstrual history: Cycles normal, LMP: 10 days back
Past history: H/o feeling mobile lump in the abdomen off and on for 1 year, no treatment taken
H/o colicky pain abdomen for 3 months

O/E
Patient seems to be in acute pain
Pulse: 110/min, BP: 110/70 mmHg
Pallor: Mild
No Lymphadenopathy
Chest/CVS: NAD

P/A: Upper abdomen soft, no organomegaly, No free fluid
Tenderness and guarding present in suprapubic region

P/V: Cx↑, uterus retroverted, normal size, cystic tender mass 6 × 8 cm palpable anterior to the uterus, both fornices free, no fullness in POD, no nodularity on PVR

Clinical impression: Twisted ovarian cyst
Plan: Urgent USG for confirmation of the diagnosis

USG: Uterus normal, ET 6 mm, cystic mass 8 × 8 cm anterior to the uterus, with intense echogenic calcified nodule and fat/fluid interface seen.

Q1. How do you diagnose twisted ovarian cyst? Using USG?

The diagnosis of the twisted ovarian cyst is clinical, with symptoms of acute colicky pain abdomen that may be associated with nausea and fever and a tender cystic pelvic mass. Location of a cyst anterior to the uterus is highly suggestive of it being an ovarian cyst as other tender masses like ectopic pregnancy, tubo-ovarian abscess or endometrioma are usually located in the adenexa. Further confirmation can be done by USG findings with Doppler flow.

Q2. What are the other causes of pain with ovarian cyst?

Ovarian cyst can present with pain if there is torsion, rupture, internal hemorrhage in the cyst.

Q3. Do you need to rule out malignancy in this case?

No, the young age of the patient along with USG findings suggestive of ovarian cyst with calcified nodule and fat/fluid interface are almost confirmatory of dermoid cyst (benign cystic teratoma).

Q4. If this cyst is detected during pregnancy, will you manage the case differently?

If we detect an ovarian cyst during pregnancy which is asymptomatic, unilocular clear cyst < 8 cm in size, we wait for spontaneous resolution of the cyst by 16 weeks as most of these are functional cysts. Ovarian cysts that are strongly suggestive of malignancy or that are larger than 8–10 cm in diameter, are symptomatic, or are at an increased risk for torsion (as with dermoid cyst), cyst rupture, or obstruction of labour are more likely to require surgical intervention. If surgery is required, it is most advantageous to perform it in the early second trimester, as the risk of spontaneous abortion during this period is lower than in the first trimester. Surgical intervention is better to avoid during the third trimester, if possible, to prevent inducing preterm delivery and to avoid technical issues in dealing with a larger uterus. But if patient presents anytime with torsion of cyst, urgent laparotomy is required. If ovarian neoplasm is detected during cesarean section, it should be removed at the same time.

Q5. Why did you specifically ask about amenorrhoea?

In reproductive age group any woman presenting with acute abdomen, ectopic pregnancy has to be ruled out. Therefore history is taken for possibility of pregnancy and if still doubtful, UPT can be done.

Few follicles seen at the periphery of the cyst. Rt ovary not seen separately, left ovary normal

Doppler studies: Twisted pedicle with altered blood flow

Impression: Twisted right ovarian dermoid cyst

Mangement: IV line and give intravenous fluids

Catheterise the bladder

Urgent Preop investigations: Hb, blood group, S. electrolytes, Urine routine

Emergency laparoscopy or laparotomy.

Q6. What are the other possibilities in this case? How would you manage them?

For answer *see* Table 14.1

Table 14.1

Clinical picture	*Diagnosis*	*Management*
Not able to pass urine Midline suprapubic cystic mass, on pressing patient may complain of sensation for urination USG: distended bladder, uterus and ovaries normal	Full bladder	Catheterize the bladder
Amenorrhoea S/S of hemoperitoneum UPT +ve Comples adenexal mass	Ruptured ectopic pregnancy	Urgent laparotomy
Tender firm mass Attached to the uterus	Torsion of subserous fibroid	Urgent laparotomy or laparoscopy with myomectomy
Occurs during pregnancy Fever, leucocytosis USG : Fibroid uterus	Fibroid uterus with red degeneration	Conservative management: Observation, Bed rest, I/V fluids and Analgesics
Vaginal discharge, fever H/O STD/PID, abortion or delivery or intrauterine procedure Leukocytosis, Raised ESR, UPT -ve USG: Complex adenexal mass, fluid may be there in POD; no fire sign	Pelvic abscess	Hospital admission Intravenous broad spectrum antibiotics to cover polymicrobial infections

15 *Gynaecological Oncology*

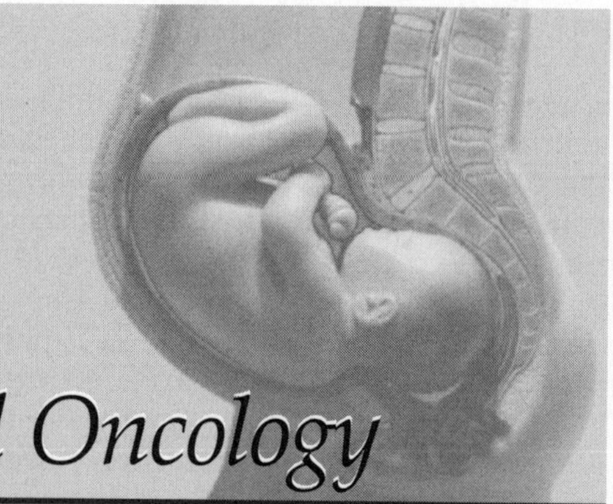

CASE 15A HIGH GRADE SQUAMOUS INTRAEPITHELIAL LESION (HSIL)

Mrs. ASDF

1st visit 17.02.08

A 37-year-old female P_4L_4 referred to GOPD because of HSIL on Pap smear

No h/o post-coital bleeeding, menorrhagia or vaginal discharge

M/h Regular cycles LMP 10.02.08
No h/o smoking

Family history:
No h/o genital tract or breast cancer

O/E
P/s Circumoral erosion on cervix, bleeds on touch
P/v Ut R/V, NS, fx free

Adv: Colposcopy and directed Bx

2nd visit 24.02.08

Satisfactory colposcopy with high grade lesion
HPE – CIN II
Adv: LEEP under local anaesthesia

Q1. The patient was referred to GOPD because of HSIL on Pap smear. What is Pap smear and what is HSIL? Is the patient having cancer?

Ca Cx is caused by HPV infection and begins as epithelial cell abnormalities in the transformation zone of the cervix. These premalignant lesions are present for many years before they progress to invasive cancer in some patients. Pap smear is an exfoliative cytology test that is used for screening women for premalignant intraepithelial abnormalities in asymptomatic stage so that the lesion can be treated before progression to invasive cancer.

The epithelial cell abnormalities are of different types and grades, and a widely accepted terminology for describing these abnormalities is the terminology of Bethesda system (Box 15.1). HSIL stands for high grade squamous intraepithelial lesion and is part of the TBS terminology.

For taking a Pap smear, an Ayre's spatula is fixed inside the external cervical os and rotated through 360° to scrape the entire transformation zone of cervix. The specimen of epithelial cells thus obtained is smeared on a slide and fixed immediately in 95% ethanol.

Box 15.1: Epithelial Cell Abnormalities (Terminology of Bethesda System-2001)

- Squamous cell
  - Atypical squamous cell (ASC)
    - Of undetermined significance (ASC-US)
    - Cannot exclude HSIL (ASC-H)
  - Low grade squamous intraepithelial Lesion (LSIL)
    - Encompassing HPV/CIN I
  - High grade squamous intraepithelial lesion (HSIL)
    - Encompassing CIN 2 and CIN 3
  - Squamous cell carcinoma
- Glandular cells
  - Atypical glandular cells (AGC) (Specify endocervical, endometrial or not otherwise specified)
  - Atypical glandular cells, favour neoplasia (Specify endocervical or non otherwise specified)
  - AIS (Adenocarcinoma in situ)
- Adenocarcinoma

Q2. In the answer to the previous question, you have referred to the transformation zone. What is it?

The cervix is covered by two types of epithelium, stratified squamous Epithelium (ectocervix) and columnar epithelium (endocervix), which meet at the squamo-columnar junction. During childhood and perimenarche, it is located at, or very close to, the external os. After puberty and during the reproductive period the cervix enlarges and the endocervical canal elongates. This leads to the eversion of the columnar epithelium onto the ectocervix, particularly on the anterior and posterior lips, resulting in ectropion or ectopy. Thus, the squamo-columnar junction is located in the ectocervix, far away from the external os during the reproductive years and pregnancy. When everted columnar epithelium is exposed to the acidic vaginal environment, this leads to the destruction and eventual replacement of the columnar epithelium by the newly formed metaplastic squamous epithelium. As a woman passes through her reproductive life to the perimenopusal age group, the location of the squamocolumnar junction progressively starts moving on the ectocervix towards the external os due to this metaplasia. The transformation zone is the area of the cervix where the columnar epithelium has been replaced and/or is being replaced by the metaplastic squamous epithelium. With the naked eye, one can identify the inner border of the transformation zone by tracing the squamocolumnar junction and the outer border by locating the distal most nabothian cysts (if present) or crypt openings (usually visible under magnification), Almost all cervical neoplasia occurs in this zone, close to the squamocolumnar junction.

Q3. You have advised colposcopy and directed Bx. Do all abnormal Pap smears need colposcopy? How does colposcopy help these patients?

All pap smears showing squamous cell abnormalities more than ASCUS and all glandular cell abnormalities need immediate colposcopy (examination in intense illumination and higher magnification). Colposcopy helps to delineate the abnormal area on cervix from which Bx can be taken. Hence, the role of colposcopy is in localizing the site of Bx and knowing the extent of lesion.

Q4. Are there any other methods for cervical screening?

Yes, there are cheaper tests like the VIA (visual inspection of cervix with acetic acid) and VILI (visual inspection of cervix with Lugol's Iodine). These are OPD procedures in which the cervix is inspected under good light after application of dilute 5% acetic acid (in VIA) and Lugol's iodine (in VILI). Any abnormal aceto-white lesion in the transformation zone (in VIA), or any non-staining pale areas (in VILI) is suggestive of premalignant condition.

On the other hand, there are costly tests like HPV-DNA testing that detects the presence of high risk oncogenic HPV infection in the genital tract. Specimen is taken in the same way as for Pap smear. At present its main use is in cases of ASCUS abnormality (atypical cells of undetermined significance) on Pap's smear to detect high risk cases for further evaluation by colposcopy.

Q5. Can we prevent HPV infection and thus prevent carcinoma cervix?

Yes, HPV vaccines are now available which can prevent infections by highly oncogenic HPV viruses (16 & 18). Three doses of vaccines (at 0, 1, 6 months) are to be administered to females between age group 9–26 years, preferably before any sexual exposure. However, since only 70% of the cervical cancers are caused by HPV (16 & 18) , not all cervical cancers can be prevented. Hence, cervical screening should continue even after vaccination.

Q6. What are the treatment options? Why LEEP has been preferred?

Moderate dysplasia (CIN II) is a precancerous lesion and one-third of them progress to invasive cancer. For treatment one can use ablative methods, e.g. cryotherapy or LASER ablation or excisional methods like LEEP or cold knife conisation. In both types of therapy, it is important to treat the whole of transformation zone irrespective of size of lesion. Excisional method has been preferred here because it provides tissue for HPE and because LEEP is cheap, cost effective, safe and efficacious. The results of cryotherapy and LEEP are the same. While using cryotherapy, the lesion should be fully visible, i.e. it should be localized to ectocervix with no extension to endocervix.

Q7. Is cervical cancer the only cancer in females for which routine screening is recommended?

No. apart from cervical cancer screening, routine screening is also recommended for breast cancer. Also, at menopause, women at average risk should be informed about the risks and symptoms of endometrial cancer and strongly encouraged to report any unexpected bleeding or spotting to their physicians.

Q8. What are the screening recommendations for breast cancer?

Beginning at 40 years of age annual screening for breast cancer should be done by:

1. Clinical breast examination by a physician and
2. Screening mammography.

   Between the age of 20 and 40 years a woman should have clinical breast examination every 3 years and can do self breast examination. She should report to a health personnel whenever she notes any change in her breasts.

Q1. In the above cases, is the reproductive history (P_5L_5) significant?

Endometrial Ca occurs more commonly in nulliparous women while Ca Cx is commoner in multiparous women.

Q2. Why has Pap smear not been done in this case?

Pap smear is a screening test done in cases of normal-looking cervix without any focal lesion. It has no role in this case where the cervical growth has all the features of malignancy, i.e. it is hard, friable, bleeds on touch and fixed (parametrial infiltration). Hence, we directly take the Bx and do histopathology to establish the definitive diagnosis.

Q3. What are the characteristic s/s of cervical carcinoma?

The *cardinal symptoms* are:

1. Vaginal discharge, which may be blood stained;
2. Bleeding P/V, which may be postcoital or intermenstrual;
3. Late symptoms like neurogenic pain due to nerve involvement, and cachexia. The *cardinal signs* are that the cervix is hard, immobile or fixed, friable, and bleeds on touch.

Q4. What investigations are necessary for the staging of Ca Cx?

The FIGO staging for carcinoma cervix (FIGO: International federation of gynecology and obstetrics) is largely clinical and its most important part is pelvic examination, particularly, rectovaginal examination. Although radiological studies (CT/MRI) tell us about lymph node spread and parametrial infiltration, they are not mandatory in FIGO staging. If there is parametrial spread, IVP or CT scan with contrast will detect if there is

CASE 15B CARCINOMA CERVIX

Mrs. X, 55 year, P_5L_5
C/o irregular bleeding per vaginum–1 month
H/o blood stained vaginal discharge–2 mth
H/o post coital bleeding +ve since 6 months

M/H
Menopausal for 8 years
Menarche – 11 years
Age at 1st coitus – 18 years

O/E
Average built
BP 110/80 mmHg
Breast – NAD
P/s – Cx replaced by growth, bleeds on touch, Vagina healthy.
P/v – Cx replaced by hard, friable growth Uterus NS, R/V
P/V/R B/L parametrium indurated, short of pelvic wall, rectal mucosa free
CI: Carcinoma cervix Stage IIb

Cervical punch Bx from edge of the growth (OPD procedure)
HPE report: Keratinizing squamous cell cancer cervix.
Plan: Radiotherapy preferably chemoradiation

Investigations:

1. HMG with platelet count
2. Urine R & M
3. LFT
4. KFT
5. X-ray Chest PA view
6. USG Kidneys/IVP (hydronephrosis due to urethral obstruction indicates stage III cancer cervix) or CT scan pelvis for parametrial extension, kidneys, and para-aortic lymph nodes

evidence of urethral occlusion or hydronephrosis. Cystoscopy or proctoscopy are warranted only if the tumor palpably encroaches upon these organs. Colposcopy can be done to assess the extent of vaginal involvement.

Radiotherapy is planned in such a way so as to give total radiation dose of 70–80 Gray to point A and 60 Gray to point B. Bladder and Rectal dosage should not exceed 60 Gray.

Point A is an imaginary point 2 cm lateral to central axis of uterus and 2 cm superior to the external os, Point B is 3 cm lateral to point A.

Q5. You have planned radiotherapy for the patient. How is it performed?

Radiotherapy is a combination of external beam teletherapy to treat the regional lymphnodes and to decrease the tumor volume, and brachytherapy delivered by intracavitary applicators or interstitial implants to provide a treatment boost to the central tumor. Recent studies have shown better results with chemoradiation than radiation alone.

Brachytherapy (brachy-means short-distance) is also called internal radiotherapy. It involves precise placement of radiation sources directly at the site of the cancerous tumour and therefore, exposure to radiation of healthy tissues further away from the sources is reduced and the tumour can be treated with very high doses of localised radiation. Another advantage is that even if the patient moves, the radiation sources retain their correct position in relation to the tumour. In teletherapy or external beam radiotherapy (EBRT), high-energy X-rays are directed at the tumour from outside the body.

Q6. Does surgery have any role in these cases?

Radial hysterectomy is considered as an option for stage I and IIa where uterus, cervix, and upper one-third of vagina are removed along with bilateral parametrial and pelvic lymphadenectomy. RT and surgery have equal cure rates in early disease. Neoadjuvant chemotherapy can be used in Stage Ib2 (bulky cancer) to decrease the size of tumor before surgery.

Advantages of surgery in early disease

- Can conserve ovary in young age
- Get specimen for HPE
- Patient's psychology–disease is out and therefore patient feels cured
- Adequate length of vagina is saved
- Avoids side effects of radiotherapy.

Disadvantage: Primary morbidity, i.e. fistula (1–2%), primary hemorrhage, Pulmonary embolism, Febrile morbidity, lymphocyst and bladder dysfunction.

Comparison of Surgery *vs* Radiotherapy for Early stages Carcinoma Cervix

	Surgery	*Radiotherapy*
Survival	85%	85%
Serious complications	Urological fistulas (1–2%)	Intestinal and urinary strictures and fistulas (1.4–5.3%)

Q7. How often does cervical carcinoma present premenopausally?

The average age at diagnosis of cervical cancer is 51, but its incidence is increasing in young women, so that nearly half the patients with it are now in premenopausal age.

Q1. What are the common causes of PMB?

PMB is an alarming symptom and calls for evaluation without delay to rule out genital tract malignancy as about 20% cases of postmenopausal bleeding are due to cancer. PMB can also be due to benign conditions, e.g., senile cervicovaginitis, cervical tuberculosis, tubercular pyometra, forgotten foreign body like pessary, anticoagulant therapy, or withdrawal of HRT.

Q2. You have mentioned withdrawal of HRT as a cause of PMB. When and why is HRT withdrawn?

Women often do not understand the importance of regularity in taking HRT (or herbal medicines with estrogenic action) or the necessity of informing the doctor when they decide to discontinue it. Such women are alarmed when they have vaginal bleeding as they do not realize it to be the consequence of stopping HRT. Hence, it is important to ask specifically for discontinuation of any medicine.

Q3. Mrs. X had bleeding P/V 10 years after her menopause and was diagnosed as a case of PMB. Would the diagnosis be the same if the bleeding occurred 6 months after menopause?

No, PMB is defined as bleeding from genital tract occurring at least 1 year after cessation of menstruation. If the bleeding occurs before 1 year after last menstruation, it could be a resumption of normal menstruation. Around this time, the bleeding should normally become progressively lighter and spaced farther apart. Menopause is essentially a retrospective diagnosis made after 1 year of last menstruation, and it is only after one year that any bleeding is called as postmenopausal bleeding.

CASE 15C ENDOMETRIAL CARCINOMA

Mrs. X, 60 years, $P_{1+0+0+1}$

1st visit 09.01.08

C/o

Bleeding P/V – 14 days

No h/o foul-smelling or blood stained vaginal discharge

No h/o post-coital bleeding

No h/o receiving anticoagulants or HRT

Menstrual history

Menarche – 11 years

Menopause at 50 years

No h/o diabetes or hypertension or tuberculosis

No family h/o colon, breast, ovary or similar malignancy

O/E

Obesity +

Wt – 90 kg

BP 120/80 mmHg

Breast NAD

P/A NAD

P/S Cx and vagina healthy, bleeding through os present

P/V Ut R/V, bulky, mobile and bilateral fornices free

P/V/R Rectal mucosa free

No induration in the parametrium

Adv

- Pap smear taken
- TVS (transvaginal ultrasonography)
- Blood investigations Hb, Blood sugar F and PP

Urine R and M

2nd visit 10.01.08

TVS and Pap smear–normal, patient reassured.

If recurrent episodes of PMB or heavy bleeding: Further evaluation by hysteroscopy and directed endometrial Bx or fractional curettage or

Pap smear – normal

TVS shows abnormality of endometrium:

- ET (endometrial thickness) >4–5 mm or is irregular or fluid in cavity

Adv:

Endometrial sampling by:

Hysteroscopy and directed endometrial Bx or endometrial aspiration biopsy or fractional curettage.

3rd visit 17.01.08

HPE: Endometrial cancer–adenocarcinoma well differentiated

- CT/MRI pelvis and abdomen
- PAC investigations
- 2 unit blood to be arranged

Plan: Surgical staging with TAH & BSO and sampling of pelvic and para-aortic lymph nodes with peritoneal cytology.

Q4. In the history of present illness, you have ruled out, among others, foul-smelling or blood-stained vaginal discharge. Why is that important?

These signs and symptoms are suggestive of advanced cervical malignancy.

Q5. Is it important to ask about the age of menarche?

Yes, early menarche and late menopause are high risk factors for endometrial carcinoma.

Q6. In the h/o past illness, we ask about diabetes, hypertension and tuberculosis. Of course, PMB can be due to tubercular pyometra, but why is it important to ask about diabetes and hypertension?

Diabetes, hypertension and obesity are risk factors for endometrial carcinoma. The corpus cancer syndrome comprises diabetes, hypertension and obesity with endometrial cancer.

Q7. Why is noting the weight important? Are you looking for a low weight that is suggestive of malignancy?

No, basically I am recording the degree of obesity because obesity is a risk factor for endometrial malignancy.

Q8. Do you examine the breast to rule out malignancy? Does it tend to coexist with PMB?

Clinical breast examination is done on every woman after 30 years to screen for malignancy. This is not related to PMB (Refer to guidelines for screening breast cancer case 15A, Q. 8).

Q9. The P/V examination reveals the uterus to be retroverted, mobile and with bilateral fornices free. Do these observations influence your diagnosis?

No, these are normal findings. A normal-sized uterus can harbor malignancy. If it is fixed and parametrial are thickened, it is more likely to be a case of cervical cancer.

Q10. You have mentioned that either endometrial aspiration biopsy can be done alone or can be combined with hysteroscopy. When will you do only endometrial biopsy? When are both necessary? Are other investigations necessary?

In all cases of postmenopausal bleeding endometrial sampling should be done to rule out endometrial malignancy. *Endometrial biopsy* is an OPD procedure which does not require anesthesia or cervical dilatation. It is done using endometrial curette (specially designed for the purpose) with which 1–2 strips of endometrial tissue are taken (usually near the cornual ends from side walls). The limitations of the procedure is that only a small area of the cavity is sampled. The procedure is done in cases of infertility (to detect ovulation and to detect endometrial tuberculosis) and in cases of dysfunctional uterine bleeding (to see if the endometrium is hyperplastic, proliferative or secretory). Since hormonal changes affect the entire endo-metrium, inferences drawn from a limited sample is reasonably correct. However, the same is insufficient in cases of suspected endometrial carcinoma because carcinomatous changes are focal and the entire endometrium needs to be sampled. Hence, in endometrial malignancies, an *endometrial 'aspiration' biopsy* is done. With newer instruments for taking biopsy, the sensitivity of detecting endometrial cancer is quite high. The device most commonly used today is the Pipelle canula: It is a plastic syringe that is inserted in the uterine cavity. The plunger is withdrawn and negative pressure sucks in endometrial tissue into the canula. Office endometrial biopsy can be the initial diagnostic procedure of choice due to its convenience, accuracy, safety and low cost. However, in up to half the cases, the sample is inadequate or it may not be possible to perform procedure without anesthesia. A positive test is more reliable for diagnosing the disease than a negative test is for ruling it out. As these canulas are costly and not available in our hospital, endometrial aspiration biopsy is not commonly done.

The best procedure for endometrial carcinoma is *hysteroscopy and directed biopsy*. With the hysteroscope, we are able to see the whole of the endometrial surface and any abnormal area is sampled during the procedure. Hysteroscopy is also useful in vaginal bleeding for detecting benign lesions like polyp and submucosal fibroid.

If a hysteroscope is not available, we do a *fractional curettage sampling* of the whole uterine cavity. This is done in the OT under local, regional or general anesthesia. During this procedure, endocervical curettings are taken (to detect endocervical cancer) and sent for histopathology. The cervix is then dilated with Hegar's dilators, endometrial curette is introduced in the uterine cavity, and the entire endometrium is curetted systematically. Being a blind procedure, usually less than half of the uterine cavity gets sampled. Hence, hysteroscopy-directed biopsy is preferable.

Q11. Why did you advise TVS for investigating PMB?

In a case of postmenopausal bleeding, ultrasonic evaluation of endometrium using TVS (transvaginal sonography) is an important non-invasive method of excluding endometrial cancer. It is usually the first line of investiga-tions. If TVS shows endometrial abnormality, i.e. irregular endometrium or thick endo-metrium ET >4–5 mm or fluid in endometrial cavity, it needs further evaluation. If TVS is normal, the patient can be reassured. But if bleeding persists or recurrent episodes of PMB occur, then also she needs further evaluation by hysteroscopy or fractional curettage.

Q12. After establishing the diagnosis of endometrial cancer, you advised CT/MRI Pelvis and abdomen. Why?

Once the histopathology reveals endometrial cancer, we would like to know the histological type and staging of the malignancy. Pre-operative staging is made possible to some extent by TVS since it can detect myometrial invasion but the X-ray chest and MR/CT of pelvis and abdomen are required to know the spread of tumor to pelvic and para-aortic lymph nodes. Preoperative staging is however optional and more often, the same is done during laparotomy. Like the histological type of the malignancy, its staging too influences the course of subsequent chemotherapy or radiotherapy.

Q13. What is the recommended management of endometrial cancer?

The primary modality of treatment is surgery, i.e. TAH with B/L SO with peritoneal cytology and pelvic and para-aortic lymph node sampling. Postoperative radiotherapy is given to high-risk cases and patients with +ve pelvic or para-aortic lymph nodes. Chemotherapy and hormonal therapy have role in advanced disease.